ARTHUR WANG

Everyday Pharmacology: How Drugs Affect Your Body and Mind

First published by Arthur Wang 2024

First edition

ISBN: 978-0-9826347-3-8

This book was professionally typeset on Reedsy.
Find out more at reedsy.com

Contents

Introduction

Obtaining prescription drugs post-visit to a doctor has become routine for many nowadays, as it's ingrained in the belief that medication effectively resolves medical issues. However, some individuals may be driven by psychological factors to seek prescriptions, even when unnecessary. On the other hand, some strongly resist medication, citing worries about side effects or a preference for exploring alternative options.

To optimize the benefits and minimize potential side effects of medication, it's imperative to deepen our understanding of how drugs interact with our bodies. While numerous drugs may address similar conditions, one may be more suitable than another for a particular individual.

The field of pharmacology, exploring how drugs affect the body, may appear daunting to laypersons. This book aims to demystify pharmacology for everyday readers, presenting complex concepts in a clear and accessible manner. Enhanced comprehension of drug interactions empowers individuals to advocate for themselves effectively and facilitates better communication with healthcare providers. Moreover, it might reveal other medication choices beyond the ones first recommended. However, it's crucial to underscore that the information provided in this book should not substitute consultation with a qualified medical professional. Always seek guidance from a healthcare provider before making any decisions regarding medication.

1

Chapter 1: Quick Understanding on Pharmacology

Welcome to "Quick Understanding on Pharmacology." In this section, I'll simplify complex drug concepts, making pharmacology accessible to all. By the time you've finished a third of the book, you'll be amazed at how easy it is to grasp. Stick to the sequential reading for maximum benefit and use this section as your go-to reference in the future. Let's dive in!

How a drug is born?

Substances utilized for treating illnesses are commonly referred to as drugs. As new applications for existing drugs are discovered or new drugs are developed, the list of available medications undergoes periodic updates. In the United States, the average time it takes for a new drug to receive approval from the FDA is approximately 10 to 12 years. This process can be broken down into several stages, including pre-clinical testing and three phases of clinical trials. The FDA aims to review and act on at least 90% of New Drug Applications (NDAs) for standard drugs no later than 10 months after the applications are received. The review goal is six months for priority drugs.

As for the cost, developing a new drug is a costly endeavor. The cost of bringing a new drug to market, from drug discovery through clinical trials to approval, typically ranges from hundreds of millions to billions of U.S. dollars. In an analysis of the drug development costs for 98 companies over a decade, the average cost per drug developed and approved by a single-drug company was $350 million. For companies that approved between eight and 13 drugs over 10 years, the cost per drug went as high as $5.5 billion. However, these figures can vary widely depending on the complexity of the drug and the length of the development process. Additionally, post-approval trials, which are sometimes mandated by the FDA as a condition of approval, are conducted; these are known as Phase 4 Trials or Post-Marketing Surveillance Trials.

The Process of New Drug Development

Drug Discovery

Synthesis, Development & Screening: 2-10 years

Pre-Clinical Testing

Lab and Animal Testing: 3-5 years

(Phase I ~ Phase III: 3 -5 year)

Phase I

Determine safety and dosage

Phase II

Assess efficacy and side effects

Phase III

Monitor efficacy and adverse reactions to long-term use

NDA (New Drug Application) Filling: 1-3 years

FDA Review and Approval

Phase IV

Post-marketing Studies and product surveillance: 4-10 years

The journey of a drug from conception to arrival on pharmacy shelves is a complex and lengthy process involving multiple steps and rigorous testing. In recent years, the landscape of drug discovery has been revolutionized by the integration of artificial intelligence (AI) technology. Through sophisticated algorithms and machine learning techniques, AI has accelerated the process of identifying potential drug candidates and predicting their efficacy with unprecedented speed and accuracy. By analyzing vast datasets of biological and chemical information, AI algorithms can identify patterns and relationships that traditional methods might overlook, leading to the discovery of novel medications and treatments for a wide range of diseases. This symbiotic relationship between AI and drug discovery holds promise for faster, more efficient development of life-saving medications, ushering in a new era of innovation in healthcare.

Potency and Efficacy

A drug's effects can be assessed based on its strength (potency) or effectiveness (efficacy). Potency refers to the quantity of drug (typically measured in milligrams) required to elicit a specific effect, such as pain relief or blood pressure reduction. For example, if 5 milligrams of drug A alleviates pain to the same degree as 10 milligrams of drug B, then drug A is considered twice as potent as drug B.

Potency and efficacy are two important concepts to understand when it comes to pharmacology and how drugs affect the body and mind. Potency refers to the strength of a drug, or how much of a drug is needed to produce a specific effect. A drug with high potency will produce a desired effect at a lower dose than a drug with low potency. This is important to consider when taking medications, as a drug that is too potent can have harmful side effects.

On the other hand, efficacy refers to the ability of a drug to produce a desired effect. A drug with high efficacy will produce a strong effect, even at low doses. Understanding the efficacy of a drug is crucial for health- conscious individuals, nurses, patients, and alternative medicine practitioners, as it can help determine the most effective treatment for a particular condition.

When it comes to choosing a medication, it's important to consider both potency and efficacy. A drug with high potency but low efficacy may not be the best choice, as it may require higher doses to achieve the desired effect. Conversely, a drug with high efficacy but low potency may be more effective at lower doses, reducing the risk of side effects.

In everyday pharmacology, understanding the concepts of potency and efficacy can help individuals make informed decisions about their health and well-being. By working closely with healthcare providers and pharmacists, patients can ensure they are receiving the most effective treatment for their specific needs. Additionally, alternative medicine practitioners can use this knowledge to provide safe and effective treatments to their clients. Overall, a solid understanding of potency and efficacy is essential for anyone interested in how drugs affect the body and mind.

Four Major Effects of Drug

In the world of pharmacology, it is important to understand the various effects that drugs can have on the body and mind. There are four major effects of drugs that everyone should be aware of, whether you are a health-conscious individual, nurse, patient, alternative medicine practitioner, or any other health worker.

1. **Therapeutic Effects:** One of the main reasons why drugs are prescribed is to produce a therapeutic effect. This means that the drug is intended to treat a specific condition or disease, such as lowering blood pressure, reducing pain, or fighting infection. Understanding the therapeutic effects of a drug is crucial for ensuring that it is being used correctly and effectively.
2. **Side Effects:** Along with their therapeutic effects, drugs can also produce side effects. These are unintended or undesirable effects that occur as a result of taking a medication. Side effects can range from mild to severe and may affect different parts of the body, such as the digestive system, nervous system, or skin. It is important to be aware of potential side effects when taking any medication and to report them to your healthcare provider if they occur.
3. **Drug Interactions:** Drugs can interact with each other in various ways, affecting how they are absorbed, metabolized, or eliminated from the body. Drug interactions can lead to decreased effectiveness of a medication, increased risk of side effects, or even toxicity. It is important to inform your healthcare provider about all the medications, supplements, and herbal remedies you are taking to avoid

potentially harmful drug interactions.

4. **Dependence and Addiction:** Some drugs have the potential to cause physical or psychological dependence, leading to addiction. Dependence occurs when the body becomes accustomed to the presence of a drug and requires it to function normally. Addiction is a complex brain disorder characterized by compulsive drug seeking and use, despite harmful consequences. It is important to be aware of the addictive potential of certain drugs and to use them only as prescribed by a healthcare provider.

By understanding these four major effects of drugs, you can make informed decisions about your healthcare and ensure safe and effective use of medications. Remember to always consult with a healthcare provider before starting or stopping any medication, and to report any concerning symptoms or side effects promptly.

Understanding Drug Mechanisms: From Cells to Organs

1. **Understand Drug Effects on the Cellular Level**

Cells are intricate machines with numerous receptors dotting their surface, similar to the buttons on a car dashboard. When a substance or drug binds to a specific receptor, it acts like pressing one of these buttons. This interaction sets off a chain reaction within the cell, resembling the relay activity or cascade pathway initiated by pressing a button on the dashboard. Each binding event triggers a specific action within the cell, influencing its behavior and functionality.

2. **Understanding Drug Functionality: Enzyme Inhibition**

Within the realm of cellular activities, biochemical reactions often rely on intermediary agents, with enzymes serving as the facilitators, guiding reactions from point A to point B. In this context, drugs function by temporarily or permanently inhibiting these enzymes, effectively halting the reaction or pathway they oversee. Consequently, the intended cellular process is obstructed and fails to proceed. The degree of inhibition is contingent upon the concentration of the drug substance present. For instance, if there are 100 molecules of enzyme X and 50 molecules of the drug, the activity of enzyme X will be reduced by 50%. This mechanism underscores the pivotal role of enzymes in cellular processes and highlights how drugs can modulate these activities.

3. **Understanding Anti-Metabolites Drug Impact on DNA Synthesis**

Anti-metabolite drugs are primarily designed to target cancerous cells by disrupting the synthesis of DNA or RNA, effectively halting their ability to proliferate or grow. For instance, folic acid, also known as folate, plays a crucial role as a cofactor, a helper substance that assists in various cellular processes, including DNA replication and purine biosynthesis. Purines are essential components that make up the DNA strand.

Certain drugs, known as folic acid antagonists, such as methotrexate and 5-fluorouracil (5-FU), interfere with the enzymatic pathways involved in nucleic acid biosynthesis by substituting for folic acid. This substitution disrupts the production pathway, ultimately leading to the demise of cancer cells. When a substance is classified as an antagonist to a specific receptor, it means that the substance can bind to the receptor but does not trigger a signal. Thus, it inactivates the receptor. In the case of folic acid antagonists, they inhibit enzymes involved in DNA synthesis, effectively shutting down the production pathway and killing cancer cells. Such mechanisms highlight the targeted approach of anti-metabolite drugs in combating cancer by interfering with essential cellular processes.

4. **Understanding Drug Effects by Altering Organ Chemistry**

Certain drugs have the ability to modify the chemistry of specific organs, thereby reversing the illness condition within the patient's body. For instance, antacids serve to increase the pH level within the stomach, effectively alleviating discomfort caused by acid reflux. Through this mechanism, antacids neutralize excess acid, providing relief from symptoms. This exemplifies how drugs can induce both physical and chemical changes within organs to restore health and well-being.

Receptors

Receptors are key players in the field of pharmacology, as they are the molecules in our bodies that interact with drugs to produce their effects. These specialized proteins are found on the surface of cells throughout our bodies and are responsible for transmitting signals from the outside world to the inside of our cells.

For health-conscious individuals, nurses, patients, and alternative medicine practitioners, having a basic understanding of how receptors work can help them make informed decisions about their health and the medications they take. By understanding which receptors are targeted by different drugs, individuals can better understand the potential side effects and interactions that may occur. The role of receptors is crucial in elucidating how drugs interact with cells to achieve their therapeutic effects. While only a limited number of receptors have been identified to date, they serve as virtual structures that aid in comprehending drug mechanisms within the body. Receptors can be broadly categorized into two main types based on their interaction with drugs: activators and blockers. Activator receptors enhance the production of specific biochemical pathways, whereas blocker receptors inhibit the production of specific metabolites.

It's important to note that receptors aren't solely located on the exterior of cells; they can also be found within the cell itself. For instance, fat-soluble drugs like steroids can traverse cell membranes, which are composed of fat-soluble substances. Conversely, water-soluble drugs face difficulty entering cells directly. Therefore, it's postulated that receptors or transporters facilitate the entry of these substances into cells. This concept of receptors provides valuable insights into how drugs may exert their effects within the body.

There are three primary types of receptors situated outside of cells that govern the entry or action of drugs.

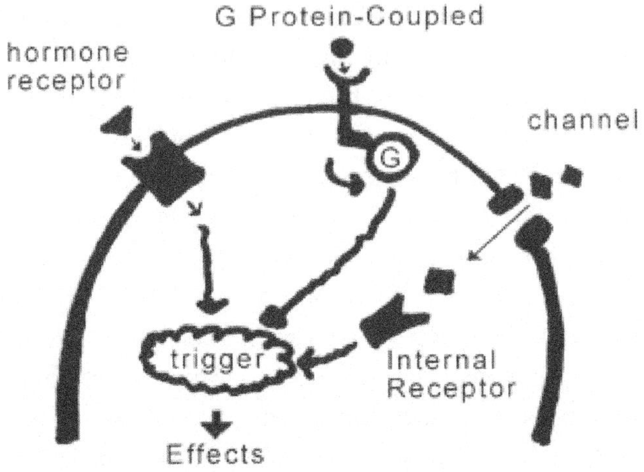

1. Channels

Cell membranes host a variety of channels, including Chloride (Cl-), Potassium (K+), Sodium (Na+), Calcium (Ca 2+), and Proton channels. Drugs may interact with specific receptors, directly or indirectly leading to the opening of certain channels. Upon activation, these channels allow ions to flow into the cell, initiating biochemical pathways that produce the desired therapeutic effect.

2. G Protein-Coupled Receptor (GPCR)

Many drugs leverage G protein-coupled receptors (GPCRs) to enact their therapeutic effects. Conceptually, GPCRs can be likened to light switches, capable of being toggled on and off by altering their configuration. By binding to the receptor, drugs induce conformational changes that initiate cellular processes, akin to flicking a light switch. Conversely, the process can be reversed or deactivated under specific conditions. For instance, chronic myelogenous leukemia (CML) arises when a GPCR known as tyrosine kinase remains in the "ON" position, leading to uncontrolled growth of cancer cells. (Further exploration of this topic will be provided in the section on Cancer Medications.)

3. Hormone Receptors

Hormone receptors play a crucial role in either triggering the release or blocking the release of specific hormones. Molecules that trigger these receptors are termed agonists, while those that block or inhibit hormone production are termed antagonists, as discussed in Anti-Metabolites Drug.

3.1. Acetylcholine Receptors (ACh)

The body hosts two primary types of acetylcholine receptors: nicotine acetylcholine receptors (nAChRs) and muscarine acetylcholine receptors (mAChRs). These receptors are named based on the molecules they bind to; for instance, the nACh receptor, also known as the nicotine receptor, was named after nicotine, which binds to it. Nicotine mimics the action of acetylcholine, a naturally occurring substance, by binding it to this receptor.

3.2. Hormone Receptors in Organs

The adrenal glands, situated near the kidneys, secrete catecholamines from their adrenal medulla. These catecholamines, including dopamine, epinephrine, and norepinephrine, enter the bloodstream and target organs with adrenergic receptors on their surface. Depending on the type of receptor—Alpha1, Alpha 2, Beta 1, or Beta 2—it elicits different effects on the organ. For example, activation of beta receptors increases the rate and force of contraction of the heart muscle.

3.3. Serotonin (5-Hydroxytryptamine, 5HT)

Serotonin, a type of amino acid, is predominantly found in the GI (gastrointestinal tract) (90%), platelets (9%), and nervous system (>1%). It serves as a neurotransmitter, influencing sleep, mood, intestinal movements, and cognitive function. In the bloodstream, serotonin also regulates blood clotting.

Synapses

Synapses serve as crucial junctions in mediating the effects of drugs on both our body and mind. These microscopic gaps between nerve cells facilitate communication, allowing messages to travel from one cell to another. Acting as spaces or junctions between two terminals of a neuron and its receiving cell, synapses rely on neurotransmitters as carriers to transmit signals.

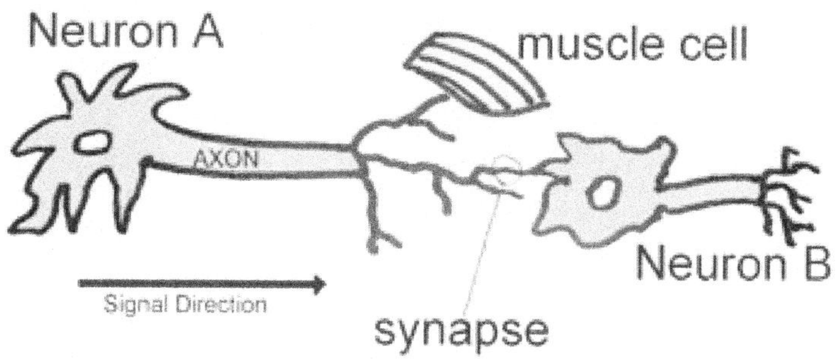

Analogous to hops in internet communication, synapses facilitate the transmission of signals to target cells, which can include muscle fibers or other neurons. Drugs exert their influence directly on synapses or indirectly by modulating the production of specific neurotransmitters. Upon nerve cell activation, neurotransmitters are released into the synapse and bind to receptors on the receiving cell, eliciting a response. Drugs can either enhance or inhibit this process, resulting in various effects on the body and mind.

Additionally, nerve impulses are propagated via voltage-gated ion channels embedded in neuron membranes, allowing action potentials to travel along axons like waves of voltage. For instance, stimulant drugs like caffeine enhance the release of neurotransmitters such as dopamine and norepinephrine, leading to heightened alertness and energy. Conversely, drugs like benzodiazepines enhance the effects of the neurotransmitter GABA, inducing a calming effect on the brain. While not all drugs directly target synapses—some, like antibiotics, act on specific bacteria or viruses, and chemotherapy drugs target cancer cells—comprehending synaptic function is integral to understanding drug mechanisms and potential side effects.

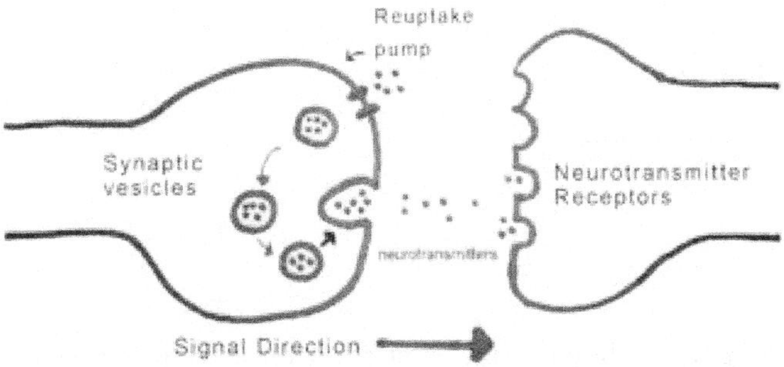

Given that synapses play a pivotal role in various conditions, gaining insight into their function enhances our understanding of how drugs can effectively interact with this area to alleviate symptoms.

Drug Dynamic Inside the human body

The interaction between drugs and the human body is a dynamic process influenced by various factors. The effectiveness of a drug depends on several elements, including dosage, individual health status, and the body's ability to metabolize and eliminate the drug. Therapeutic Drug Monitoring (TDM) assists in determining the appropriate dosage to achieve the desired therapeutic effect while avoiding toxicity. Factors contributing to the variability in drug response include genetics, age, and liver function.

Upon ingestion, drugs enter the bloodstream and travel to their target sites, where they bind to specific receptors on cells. This binding initiate biochemical reactions that produce the intended effect. However, drugs vary in their mechanisms of action – some block receptors, while others enhance their activity. Additionally, the body's ability to metabolize drugs differs among individuals, affecting drug response.

Understanding drug dynamics is crucial for individuals taking medications and healthcare professionals alike. By comprehending how drugs interact with the body, informed decisions can be made regarding medication use, potential side effects, and drug interactions. Furthermore, awareness of pharmacological principles empowers individuals to prioritize their health and well-being.

Five primary mechanisms contribute to drug dynamics:

1. **Absorption by Diffusion:** Drug molecules move from areas of high concentration to low concentration without requiring energy, akin to collecting rainwater.
2. **Absorption by Active Transport:** Some molecules, like vitamins and bile salts, require energy for active transport, resembling the process of purchasing water from a bottled water company and expending effort in the exchange
3. **Distribution:** Drugs enter the bloodstream and circulate throughout the body, analogous to goods being transported via a freeway system.
4. **Degradation:** Drugs may degrade or be destroyed through various means, including dissolution in water, pH level changes, temperature fluctuations, or enzymatic processes. This degradation process can be compared to items being discarded or recycled based on their stability

and composition. The capacity to metabolize a particular compound also varies among individuals. In the case of theophylline, heavy smokers generally display lower concentrations of this substance compared to non-smokers. This phenomenon occurs because the liver of a heavy smoker produces a greater quantity of metabolic enzymes, leading to accelerated breakdown of theophylline and consequently reduced concentrations of the compound in the bloodstream.

5. **Elimination by Kidneys and Liver:** After drugs exert their effects on the body, they are metabolized and eliminated primarily through the kidneys and liver. In the kidneys, drugs are filtered from the bloodstream and excreted through urine, while in the liver, they undergo biotransformation into metabolites that are more easily eliminated. This process ensures that drugs are efficiently removed from the body, preventing their accumulation to toxic levels. Factors such as kidney and liver function, hydration status, and urinary pH can influence the rate of drug elimination, leading to variations in drug clearance among individuals. Understanding the role of these organs in drug metabolism and elimination is vital for optimizing drug therapy and minimizing the risk of adverse effects.

The Risks of Drug Interactions and Beyond

In managing various illnesses, it's common for individuals to require multiple medications throughout the day rather than relying on a single drug. However, with each additional drug, the likelihood of experiencing side effects increases disproportionately.

Mixing drugs, whether they are prescription medications, over-the-counter remedies, or recreational substances, can yield serious consequences for both your body and mind. The interaction between different drugs can lead to unexpected outcomes, posing risks of dangerous side effects and potentially life-threatening complications.

One significant danger of combining drugs is the occurrence of drug-drug interactions. Certain medications may interact with each other, either amplifying or diminishing their effects. This can result in an overdose of one or both drugs, manifesting symptoms such as dizziness, confusion, respiratory depression, or even coma. It is imperative to seek guidance from a healthcare professional before combining medications to ensure their safety and efficacy.

Beyond drug-drug interactions, mixing drugs can also give rise to drug-food interactions. Some medications may interact with specific foods, drinks, or dietary supplements, altering their absorption, metabolism, or elimination from the body. For instance, consuming tyramine-rich foods like cheese or avocados while taking Monoamine Oxidase Inhibitors (MAOIs) can trigger a hypertensive crisis due to compromised monoamine metabolism. This underscores the importance of understanding and adhering to dietary restrictions associated with certain medications.

Moreover, the combination of drugs can impact mental health and emotional well-being. Certain drug combinations may exacerbate symptoms of anxiety, depression, or other mental health conditions. They can also impair judgment, coordination, and decision-making abilities, heightening the risk of accidents, injuries, or risky behaviors.

To safeguard your health and well-being, it's crucial to adhere to prescribed dosages and instructions for each medication. Avoid self-medication or mixing drugs without consulting a healthcare professional first. Your pharmacist, doctor, or nurse can offer valuable insights and guidance on the potential risks and benefits associated with combining different drugs.

Remember, your health is paramount, and staying informed and cautious about the effects of mixing drugs is essential. Prioritize your well-being above all else to ensure a safe and healthy lifestyle.

2

Chapter 2: Drugs that are Easy to Understand

Anti-diarrhea Medications and Diarrhea Treatment Options

Diarrhea is a common affliction that can disrupt daily life for people of all ages. In this section, we explore the various methods available for treating and handling diarrhea, focusing particularly on anti-diarrheal medications.

Anti-diarrheal drugs function by slowing down intestinal movement, affording the body more time to absorb water and nutrients from stool. This action helps alleviate symptoms such as cramping and dehydration, reducing the frequency and urgency of bowel movements.

Over-the-counter anti-diarrheal options like loperamide (Imodium) and bismuth subsalicylate (Pepto-Bismol) are widely accessible and generally effective for short-term use. However, adherence to dosage instructions is important to avoid potential side effects like constipation or bloating.

It's important to recognize that diarrhea is the body's response to an abnormal condition, often a protective mechanism to rid the intestines of harmful substances. Therefore, simply halting diarrhea doesn't address the underlying issue.

1. **Stabilizing Digestive Tracts:** Intestines house beneficial bacteria crucial for health and digestion. Probiotics, such as Bifidobacterium and Lactic Acid bacteria, help maintain optimal pH levels and inhibit harmful bacterial growth. Additionally, incorporating fermented foods rich in probiotics, such as yogurt, kefir, and kimchi, can further support gut health.
2. **Bowel Movement Inhibition:** Loperamide hydrochloride can temper exaggerated intestinal movements, slowing bowel movements by interacting with proteins in the intestinal lining.
3. **Anti-Inflammatory:** Bismuth, for instance, can form water-insoluble compounds with proteins, effectively insulating inflamed intestinal cells.
4. **Absorption:** Drugs like aluminum silicate and dimethicone counter excessive water absorption or gas build-up, easing bowel movements.
5. **Regulating Bile Salt:** Agents like scopolia control overexcited parasympathetic nerve activity, reducing excessive bile salt secretion and water content.
6. **Analgesics:** Codeine phosphate blocks nerve transmissions from the parasympathetic nervous system, effectively halting diarrhea.

For those inclined towards natural remedies, herbal supplements like probiotics, ginger, and chamomile tea offer potential relief with anti-inflammatory and soothing effects on the digestive system.

However, it's essential to recognize that while anti-diarrheal medications provide temporary relief, they don't address underlying conditions causing chronic diarrhea. Persistent or severe symptoms warrant consultation with a healthcare professional for a comprehensive treatment plan. Maintaining a healthy gut microbiome is paramount for digestion and overall well-being. Probiotics can aid in preventing and treating diarrhea by restoring beneficial gut bacteria and rebalancing the gut microbiota.

In conclusion, anti-diarrheal medications serve as valuable tools for managing acute diarrhea episodes and alleviating uncomfortable symptoms. By understanding their mechanisms and appropriate usage, individuals can take charge of their digestive health and enhance their overall quality of life.

Gastrointestinal Stimulants: Alleviating Constipation Discomfort

Gastrointestinal stimulants represent a common class of medications utilized to alleviate constipation, a prevalent condition causing discomfort and potential pain for many individuals. Constipation occurs when the colon absorbs excessive water or when the colon muscles function improperly, leading to difficulties in passing stool.

These stimulants function by enhancing intestinal motility, facilitating the swift movement of stool through the digestive tract. This action aids in relieving constipation and fostering regular bowel movements. While often employed for short-term constipation relief, they can also address more chronic conditions.

Constipation discomfort varies among individuals, primarily stemming from excessive water absorption in the GI tract or sluggish GI tract movement. Identifying the root cause of chronic constipation is essential for effective management.

Laxatives, administered when necessary, typically act via four main methods:

Osmotic Agents and Saline Laxatives: These agents draw water into the intestinal tract, exerting pressure that stimulates muscle contraction. However, electrolyte loss or dehydration may occur as side effects. Examples include magnesium oxide, magnesium sulfate, and sodium sulfate.

Fiber Products/Bulk-Forming Agents: Such drugs augment intestinal tract volume, facilitating bowel movement. It's essential to consume ample water alongside this laxative type. Examples encompass carmellose sodium, guar gum, and Psyllium.

Stool Softeners and Lubricants: These laxatives allow fluids to blend into stool, reducing its surface tension and facilitating easier passage. An example is dioctyl sodium sulfosuccinate (DSS).

Carbohydrate Laxatives: Sorbitol, for instance, is often favored for elderly patients with compromised liver function. It functions similarly to saline laxatives and promotes gas formation within the GI tract, thereby improving bowel movement.

Laxatives Acting by Stimulation:

Stimulant Laxatives: These agents chemically prompt intestinal tract movement, acting either on the small or large intestine. For instance, Ricinus Communis Oil (Castor oil) acts on the small intestine, while bisacodyl or sodium picosulfate targets the large intestine. Numerous herbal extracts also operate at this level.

Central Nervous System Stimulant Laxatives: Pantethine, a derivative of Vitamin B5, stimulates the central nervous system to increase bowel movements.

Various gastrointestinal stimulants, such as bisacodyl, senna, and castor oil, are available, each working differently to stimulate intestinal muscles and facilitate bowel movements. It's crucial to adhere to the dosing instructions provided by healthcare providers to prevent side effects like cramping, diarrhea, or dehydration.

If experiencing constipation, consulting a healthcare provider before commencing any new medication is paramount. They can identify the underlying cause of constipation and recommend suitable treatment options, considering medications and lifestyle changes such as dietary adjustments, hydration, and regular exercise.

Gastrointestinal stimulants offer a valuable means of alleviating constipation discomfort and promoting regular bowel movements. It's important to note that intestines house beneficial bacteria crucial for health and digestion, and disruption of this balance can lead to gastrointestinal issues. Probiotics, such as Bifidobacterium and Lactic Acid bacteria, play a key role in maintaining this balance and supporting gut health. However, responsible use of gastrointestinal stimulants under healthcare provider guidance is imperative to ensure safe and effective treatment without disrupting the delicate balance of gut flora.

Anti-gout Medication

Gout, a form of arthritis characterized by intense joint pain and inflammation due to uric acid buildup in the body, can significantly impact daily life. Anti-gout medications play a crucial role in treatment plans to address this condition.

Gout is a recurrent condition arising from abnormal purine metabolism. It accumulates uric acid and crystallizes in joints, tendons, and tissues, resulting in inflammation and pain. Because it is recurrent in nature, gout necessitates categorizing anti-gout medications based on their conditions.

Purine is one of the components that make up DNA.

Purines —> hypoxanthine —> xanthine —> uric acid —> uric crystals —> Pain

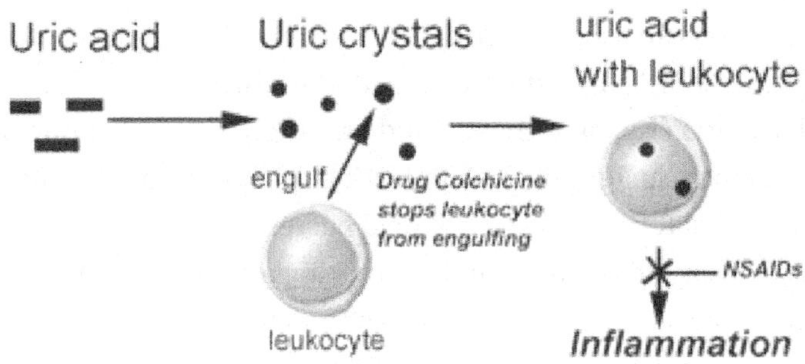

Drugs that Prevent Gout Recurrence:

Allopurinol, a common medication, inhibits the enzyme xanthine oxidase, responsible for uric acid production. By curtailing uric acid levels, allopurinol aids in preventing gout attacks. Similarly, probenecid blocks kidney function, impeding uric acid recycling to the bloodstream, and facilitating its expulsion.

However, this may elevate urine acidity, fostering kidney stone formation. To mitigate this risk, sodium hydrogen carbonate or sodium citrate may be prescribed.

Drugs that Treat Acute Gout Attacks:

Colchicine, another anti-gout medication, combats inflammation and pain during gout flare-ups. It impedes leukocyte movement by affecting microtubules, thereby alleviating inflammation caused by leukocytes engulfing deposited crystals. Although effective, colchicine may initially exacerbate pain as leukocytes release lysosomal enzymes, further inflaming tissues.

Non-steroidal anti-inflammatory drugs (NSAIDs) like naproxen or indomethacin are also employed to mitigate gout-related pain and inflammation by blocking prostaglandin-producing enzymes.

Collaboration with healthcare providers is vital for individuals with gout to identify suitable anti-gout medications tailored to their needs. Alongside medication, lifestyle modifications such as dietary adjustments, hydration, and avoiding trigger foods contribute to symptom management.

Blood-fat Reducers (Antihyperlipidemics Drugs)

Elevated levels of fats in the blood pose a significant risk factor for various cardiovascular ailments, including strokes and heart attacks. Despite the essential structural and storage roles fats play in the body, their excessive accumulation can lead to severe health complications. Unlike carbohydrates or proteins, fats necessitate substantial energy expenditure for metabolism, making them a challenge for the body to utilize efficiently. As fats accumulate in the bloodstream, they tend to adhere to blood vessel walls, causing blockages or reducing vessel flexibility. This can precipitate life-threatening conditions such as heart attacks, where the heart's oxygen supply is compromised due to blocked blood flow, or strokes, where hardened vessel walls burst under pressure, leading to blood clots.

Understanding the different types of fats present in the blood is crucial for comprehending how antihyperlipidemic drugs function.

1. Cholesterol:

Cholesterol serves as a precursor for essential bodily components such as hormones, bile acids, and fat-soluble vitamins.

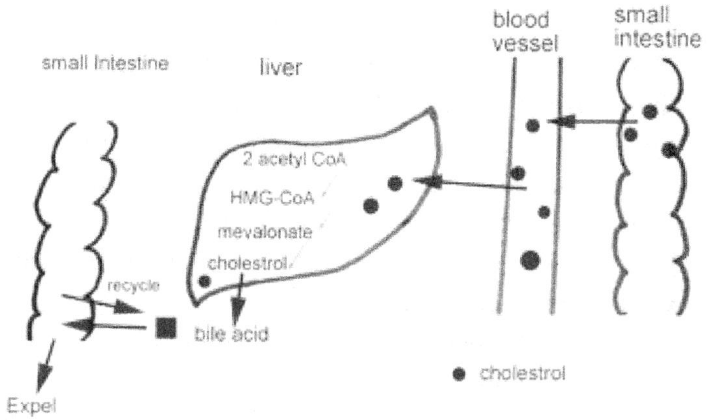

2. Lipoproteins:

Given fats' insolubility in water, lipoproteins serve as vehicles for transporting cholesterol and other fats in the bloodstream. They possess sophisticated targeting mechanisms akin to a GPS, with different types serving specific routes and destinations. Major types include chylomicrons, very-low-density lipoprotein (VLDL), intermediate-density lipoprotein (IDL), low-density lipoprotein (LDL), and high-density lipoprotein (HDL).

3. Triglycerides (TG):

Triglycerides constitute a significant portion of chylomicrons and VLDL. Elevated TG levels often correlate with higher LDL (bad cholesterol) and lower HDL (good cholesterol), indicating an increased risk of high cholesterol levels.

Distinguishing between "good" and "bad" cholesterol carriers is critical. HDL efficiently removes excess cholesterol from the bloodstream, while LDL transports cholesterol throughout the body, potentially depositing it in artery walls, leading to blockages. To help you remember, you might envision LDL as carrying an excessive number of parcels simultaneously, leading to frequent losses along the way. Consequently, LDL is often deemed detrimental. In contrast, HDL is considered beneficial because its high-density lipoprotein has the capacity to transport a greater amount of cholesterol.

Different classes of antihyperlipidemic drugs target various aspects of lipid metabolism:

1. HMG-CoA Reductase Inhibitors (Statins):

These drugs inhibit the enzyme HMG-CoA reductase, thereby reducing cholesterol production in the liver. Lower cholesterol levels prompt the liver to produce more LDL receptors, facilitating cholesterol removal from the bloodstream. Examples include pravastatin sodium, simvastatin, and atorvastatin calcium hydrate.

2. Bile Acid Sequestrants or Ion Exchange Resins:

Drugs like Colestilan and colestyramine disrupt bile acid recycling in the enterohepatic circulation, reducing cholesterol levels by increasing LDL receptor activity.

3. Probucol:

This medication prevents arterial clogging by inhibiting the oxidation of LDL cholesterol molecules, which can lead to plaque formation.

4. Cholesterol Absorption Inhibitors:

Drugs like ezetimibe prevent intestinal cholesterol absorption, leading to its excretion from the body.

5. Triglyceride-Lowering Agents:

Fibrates such as clofibrate and derivatives of nicotinic acid decrease triglyceride (TG) levels and may elevate HDL levels, consequently lowering the risk of cardiovascular complications. Examples of fibrates include clinofibrate, bezafibrate, fenofibrate, and clofibrate. Nicotinic acid derivatives like tocopherol nicotinate, nicomol, and niceritrol also exhibit similar triglyceride-lowering effects.

While antihyperlipidemic drugs effectively lower blood fat levels, they should complement healthy lifestyle practices, including diet and exercise. Collaborating with healthcare providers ensures a comprehensive approach to managing cholesterol levels, thereby mitigating cardiovascular risks effectively.

Antiglaucoma Treatment

The aqueous humor, a fluid circulating inside the eyes, serves vital functions such as providing nutrients to the lens and cornea while maintaining the eye's inner pressure to sustain its shape. However, when excess aqueous humor builds up, it can lead to heightened intraocular pressure, potentially damaging the optic nerve and causing glaucoma. Normal intraocular pressure is between 10 to 21 mm Hg, and the average is about 16.

Glaucoma manifests in two forms: open-angle (chronic) and closed-angle (acute).

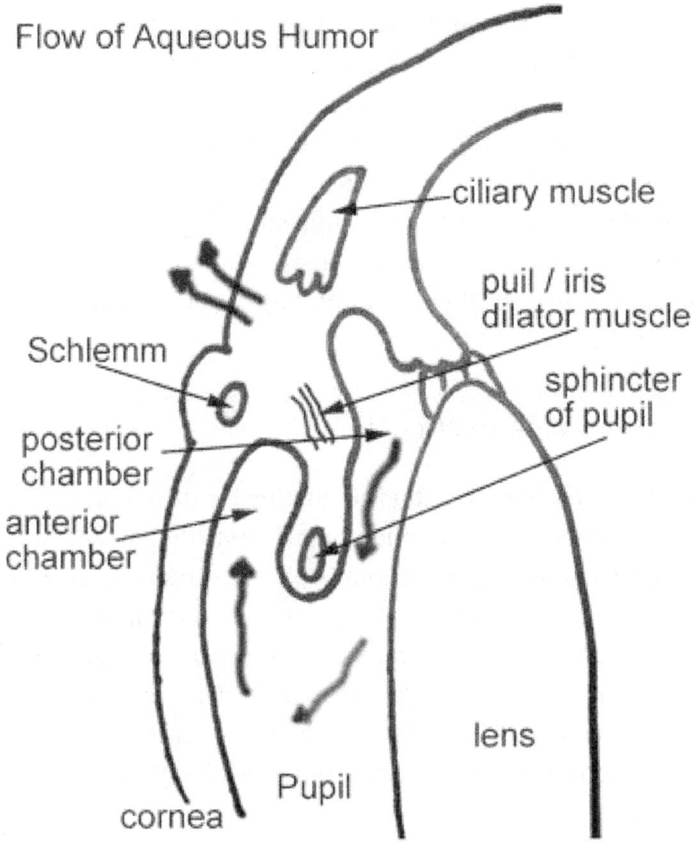

Immediate Treatment for Acute Angle Closure Glaucoma (AACG)

1. **Highly Diffusible Pressure Reducers:** Drugs like D-mannitol, isosorbide, and glycerine swiftly penetrate the eyes, extracting water from blood vessels, thus reducing

intraocular pressure and inhibiting the production of aqueous humor by the ciliary body.

2. **Carbonic Anhydrase Inhibitors:** These drugs decrease aqueous humor production by hindering carbonic anhydrase, an enzyme crucial for converting carbonic HCO3- to produce aqueous humor. Examples include acetazolamide, Neptazane, and Daranide.

Other Glaucoma Drugs for Chronic Treatment

1. **Parasympathomimetics:** These drugs increase aqueous humor outflow by expanding the Schlemm channel. Examples are pilocarpine hydrochloride, carbachol, echothiophate, and demecarium.
2. **Beta-blockers:** Originally used for hypertension, beta-blockers reduce intraocular pressure by reducing heart rate and affecting aqueous humor production. Examples include timolol maleate, carteolol hydrochloride, and betaxolol hydrochloride.
3. **Sympathomimetics:** Drugs like dipivefrin hydrochloride, an epinephrine precursor, decrease aqueous humor production and enhance fluid outflow from the eyes.
4. **Prostaglandins:** Prostaglandin analogs like isopropyl unoprostone increase aqueous humor outflow via the Schlemm channel and uveoscleral drainage.

Additionally, investigational drugs like Namenda (memantine) aim to protect the optic nerve, potentially preventing visual nerve cell shrinkage in glaucoma patients. Ginkgo biloba, an herb available over the counter, has shown promise in widening the visual field, according to studies published in

Ophthalmology.

Glaucoma is a serious eye condition that requires proper management to prevent permanent vision loss. Medications such as prostaglandin analogs, beta-blockers, and other classes of drugs help lower intraocular pressure and preserve vision. Patients should work closely with their healthcare providers to determine the most suitable treatment plan and adhere to medication regimens to maintain optimal eye health and prevent further vision damage.

Medication for Cataract

Cataracts, characterized by the clouding of the eye's natural lens, are often associated with chemical changes within the lens, which are considered part of the aging process. While the exact cause remains inconclusive, certain medications are known to have side effects that can contribute to cataract development.

Theories of Cataract Formation:

1. Free Radical Theory:

The Free Radical Theory suggests that cataracts are caused by the accumulation of free radicals in the eye. These unstable molecules can induce oxidative stress, leading to damage in the lens and eventual clouding. Factors such as exposure to ultraviolet light, ion irradiation, toxic substances, and free radicals can exacerbate this process. Glutathione, a potent antioxidant found in the lens, plays a vital role in protecting against such damage.

2. Quinoid Theory:

According to the Quinoid Theory, weakening of the eye's

ability to degrade soluble proteins can result in the formation of Quinoid substances. These substances combine with lens proteins, leading to the clouding and opacity characteristic of cataracts. Pirenoxine, a drug used in Japan for cataract patients, derivates of pyridoxine (vitamin B6), is believed to prevent Quinoid substance formation by binding to soluble proteins. Research suggests that abnormal metabolism of aromatic amino acids like tryptophan and tyrosine can lead to the development of Quinoid substances. One proposed mechanism of cataract formation involves the aggregation and cross-linking of lens proteins, leading to the formation of insoluble protein aggregates and lens opacification.

Potential Future Treatments:

1. **Salivary Gland Hormones:**

Studies have explored the use of salivary gland hormones to inhibit lens aging by reducing calcium concentration in blood vessels, potentially preventing calcium buildup in the lens and cataract formation.

2. **Sterols:**

Lanosterol, a naturally occurring steroid, has been investigated as a potential treatment for cataracts. Some research suggests that lanosterol eye drops could help clear up the clouding associated with cataracts.

Oxysterols, specifically VP1-001, are cholesterol derivatives produced via enzymatic and/or free radical oxidation. Research with mice has shown that VP1-001 can partially restore the transparency of lenses with cataracts by binding native cryAB dimers to reverse lens opacity.

Current Medications:

While surgery remains the primary treatment for cataracts, medications can help manage symptoms and slow disease progression. Eye drops containing antioxidants like vitamin C and vitamin E are commonly prescribed to reduce oxidative stress in the eye, thus slowing cataract progression and preserving vision.

In addition to antioxidants, anti-inflammatory eye drops may be used to alleviate symptoms such as inflammation, discomfort, redness, pain, and light sensitivity associated with cataracts. However, it's essential to understand that medications do not cure cataracts; surgery is often necessary to remove them and restore vision.

For individuals not yet ready for surgery or seeking alternative treatments, medications can play a valuable role in managing cataracts. Consultation with a healthcare provider is crucial to determine the most suitable treatment plan, including the use of medications, to effectively manage cataracts and preserve vision. Early intervention is key to maintaining overall eye health and preserving vision.

Non-Steroidal Anti-inflammatory Drugs (NSAIDs)

In human body, prostaglandins are versatile signaling molecules that play fundamental roles in regulating inflammation, pain, fever, smooth muscle function, and other physiological processes. They are tightly regulated in the body to maintain homeostasis. Their intricate interplay with various cellular and molecular pathways underscores their importance in health and disease. Prostaglandins play a pivotal role in pain, fever, and inflammation regulation, making them potent mediators in these physiological processes.

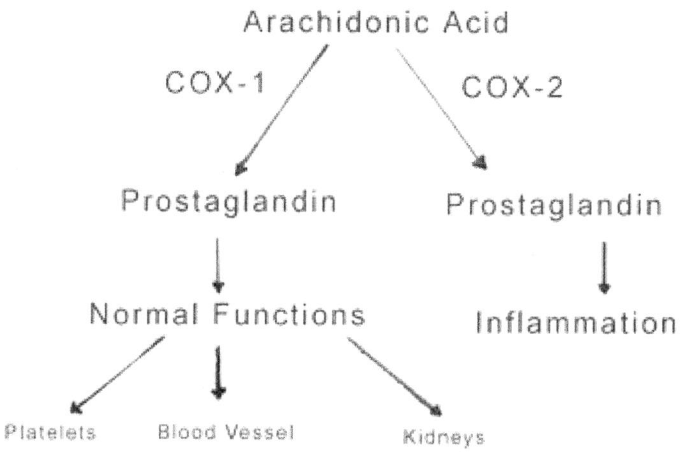

Prostaglandins exert a wide range of effects on various physiological processes in the body, including:

1. Pain:

Bradykinin is a small protein that your body produces during times of tissue injury or inflammation. Think of it as a tiny alarm bell that rings when there's damage in your body. It's part of your body's natural response to injury or inflammation. In the presence of prostaglandins, the intensity of pain amplifies.

Here's how it relates to pain:

1. **Sensitivity**: Bradykinin increases the sensitivity of the nerves responsible for pain. This means that normal pressure and temperature levels can become painful when

bradykinin is present.

2. **Inflammation**: Bradykinin promotes inflammation, which is your body's way of protecting itself from harm. It does this by causing small blood vessels to enlarge and veins to constrict, leading to leakage into capillary beds. This process can result in swelling and pain.
3. **Pain Perception**: Bradykinin plays a role in how we perceive pain. It can cause pain by directly stimulating pain-sensing nerves and by making these nerves more sensitive to stimuli that wouldn't normally be painful.

2. Fever:

The hypothalamus, acting as your body's thermostat, monitors and adjusts your temperature to maintain normal levels. During illness, increased prostaglandin production alters the hypothalamus, prompting it to raise your body's temperature setting, akin to adjusting a home thermostat. This elevation triggers heat generation by your body, inducing a fever as part of its immune defense against bacterial or viral infections. In essence, the hypothalamus, prostaglandins, and your body's temperature regulation system collaborate to produce a fever when sick.

3. Inflammation:

Inflammation is your body's natural response to injury or infection. It involves a variety of biological processes, one of which is the action of prostaglandins. Prostaglandins are hormone-like substances that your body produces primarily at sites of tissue damage or infection. They play a key role in the inflammatory response. When an injury or infection occurs, prostaglandins are released and they heighten the permeability, or 'leakiness', of your blood vessels. This increased permeability allows fluid and plasma proteins to leak out of the blood vessels and into the surrounding tissues. This leakage results in swelling, which is a classic sign of inflammation. So, in essence, prostaglandins play a crucial role in inflammation by controlling the permeability of blood vessels, leading to fluid leakage, swelling, and the overall inflammatory response. This process is part of your body's defense mechanism, helping to protect the affected area and promote healing.

4. Smooth Muscle Contraction:

Prostaglandins can either contract or relax smooth muscle tissue, depending on the specific type of prostaglandin and the target organ. For example, prostaglandins can cause uterine contractions during childbirth or relax smooth muscles in the airways to facilitate breathing.

While NSAIDs are effective for pain and inflammation relief, caution is warranted due to potential side effects such as gastrointestinal issues, kidney function impairment, and increased risk of cardiovascular events.

5. Platelet Aggregation:

Some prostaglandins promote platelet aggregation, which is essential for blood clot formation and hemostasis (stopping bleeding) following injury.

Understanding NSAIDs (Non-Steroidal Anti-Inflammatory Drugs)

Understanding how prostaglandins function in the body is pivotal for comprehending the mechanism of action, side effects, and drug selection of NSAIDs (Non-Steroidal Anti-Inflammatory Drugs).

Mechanism of Action: NSAIDs operate by curbing the production of prostaglandins. Prostaglandins are compounds within the body that spur inflammation, pain, and fever. NSAIDs can mitigate these symptoms by impeding the enzymes responsible for generating prostaglandins (COX-1 and COX-2).

Side Effects: Knowledge about prostaglandins aids in understanding the side effects of NSAIDs. Certain prostaglandins shield the stomach lining from acid; thus, when NSAIDs decrease prostaglandin production, it can result in stomach discomfort or, in severe instances, ulcers.

Drug Selection: Different NSAIDs exhibit varying degrees of selectivity for the COX-1 and COX-2 enzymes. Familiarity with these enzymes' functions and the prostaglandins they produce assists in selecting the most suitable NSAID for a particular condition.

Thus, exploring prostaglandins not only elucidates the workings of NSAIDs but also elucidates why they induce specific side effects and aids in selecting the appropriate one for distinct conditions. It is fundamental to understanding the scientific basis behind these widely utilized medications.

Aspirin, or acetylsalicylic acid, stands as a quintessential example of an NSAID. It operates by impeding prostaglandin synthesis from arachidonic acid via cyclooxygenase (COX). Two COX forms exist: COX-1 orchestrates physiological prostaglandin production, while COX-2, activated by inflammatory cells, oversees inflammation-induced prostaglandins. However, NSAIDs targeting both COX-1 and COX-2 might induce gastrointestinal discomfort due to their influence on regular digestion mediated by prostaglandins. Ongoing endeavors aim to devise drugs specifically targeting COX-2 to mitigate such adverse effects, encompassing stomach lesions and renal toxicity.

Various NSAIDs encompass acetylsalicylic acid (aspirin), meloxicam, mofezolac, etodolac, nabumetone, sulindac, diclofenac, azltoprofen, mefenamic acid, and tiaramide.

Here is a table summarizing the mechanism of action of the NSAIDs you listed, and how they relate to pain, fever, inflammation, smooth muscle contraction, and platelet aggregation:

Note: While most NSAIDs inhibit both COX-1 and COX-2 enzymes to varying degrees, some have selectivity for COX-2, which is induced during inflammation. This selectivity reduces the risk of gastrointestinal side effects associated with inhibiting COX-1, which is involved in maintaining the gastric mucosa.

It is essential to consult a healthcare provider before using NSAIDs, especially long-term or high-dose. Exploring alternative pain management strategies like acupuncture, chiropractic care, physical therapy, and dietary adjustments can also be beneficial.

Ultimately, informed decision-making and proactive healthcare approaches ensure optimal well-being.

Treating Prostate Enlargement

Prostate enlargement, also known as benign prostatic hyperplasia (BPH), is a common condition affecting men as they age. It occurs when the prostate gland, situated below the bladder and encircling the urethra, undergoes enlargement, leading to symptoms such as frequent urination, weak urine stream, and difficulty initiating or stopping urination. Although BPH typically isn't severe, it can significantly impact quality of life.

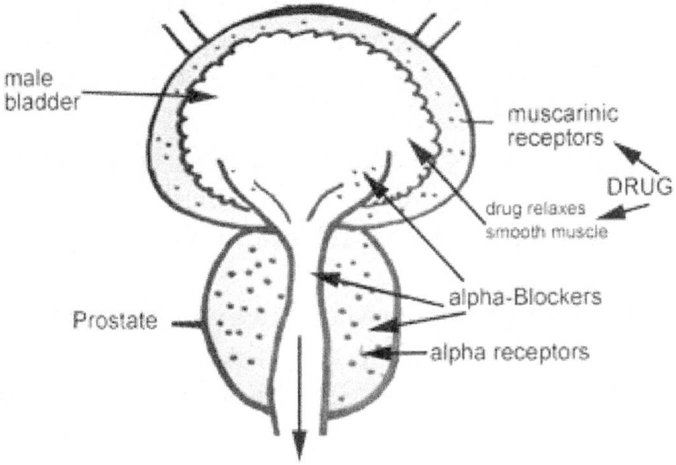

There are various treatment options for managing prostate enlargement, ranging from lifestyle changes to medications to surgical interventions. For individuals seeking natural approaches to alleviate BPH symptoms, maintaining a healthy weight, staying physically active, and avoiding bladder-irritating substances like caffeine and alcohol can be beneficial.

Medications are integral in effectively managing symptoms associated with benign prostatic hyperplasia (BPH) for many individuals. These medications target specific aspects of the condition to provide relief and improve urinary function.

Alpha-blockers:

Alpha-blockers such as tamsulosin are designed to ease the symptoms of BPH by relaxing the muscles surrounding the prostate and bladder. By doing so, they facilitate smoother urination. These drugs work by blocking alpha receptors on the cells of the urethra and bladder, leading to the widening of the urethra. Examples of alpha-blockers include tamsulosin and naftopidil.

5-alpha reductase inhibitors:

Another class of medications, known as 5-alpha reductase inhibitors, serve to reduce the size of the prostate gland over time. Drugs like finasteride fall into this category and work by inhibiting the conversion of testosterone into dihydrotestosterone (DHT), a hormone that contributes to prostate growth. In some cases, a combination of alpha-blockers and 5-alpha reductase inhibitors may be prescribed to maximize treatment efficacy.

Prostate inhibitors:

Specific medications known as prostate inhibitors target the hormonal imbalance that fuels prostate enlargement. These drugs, including chlormadione acetate and allylestrenol, address the underlying hormonal factors contributing to prostate growth, thereby helping to alleviate BPH symptoms.

Additionally, medications like flavoxate hydrochloride can enhance bladder capacity by relaxing the smooth muscle cells in the bladder wall, thereby reducing the frequency of urination.

Similarly, tolterodine tartrate works by blocking nerve impulses responsible for triggering bladder contractions, thus mitigating the urgency to urinate. As a muscarinic receptor antagonist, this drug competes for the receptor for acetylcholine, the natural neurotransmitter responsible for relaying signals in the synapse area. (See Chapter 1 for Synapses)

By targeting various aspects of BPH pathology, these medications offer tailored relief for individuals grappling with the symptoms of this common condition. In more severe cases of BPH, surgical intervention may be necessary to remove part of the prostate gland and relieve symptoms.

Procedures like transurethral resection of the prostate (TURP) or laser surgery can effectively reduce prostate size and improve urinary function.

Ultimately, the treatment approach for prostate enlargement is tailored to each individual's symptoms and preferences. It's essential for patients to discuss their options with a healthcare provider to determine the most suitable course of action for managing their BPH effectively.

3

Chapter 3: Drugs that are Understandable if you have a little more time

If you've followed along this far, you likely have a good understanding of how drugs function. Let's explore this topic and other medications available to treat commonly known illnesses.

Medication for Diabetes

Diabetes, also known as *diabetes mellitus*, is a metabolic disorder characterized by impaired glucose utilization, leading to various complications such as vision loss, kidney discomfort, and nerve damage. Insulin, a hormone produced by the pancreas, plays a crucial role in enabling cells to absorb glucose for energy production. Diabetes can occur when the pancreas fails to produce enough insulin (Type 1 diabetes) or when cells do not respond effectively to insulin (Type 2 diabetes). Gestational diabetes is another form that can affect pregnant women.

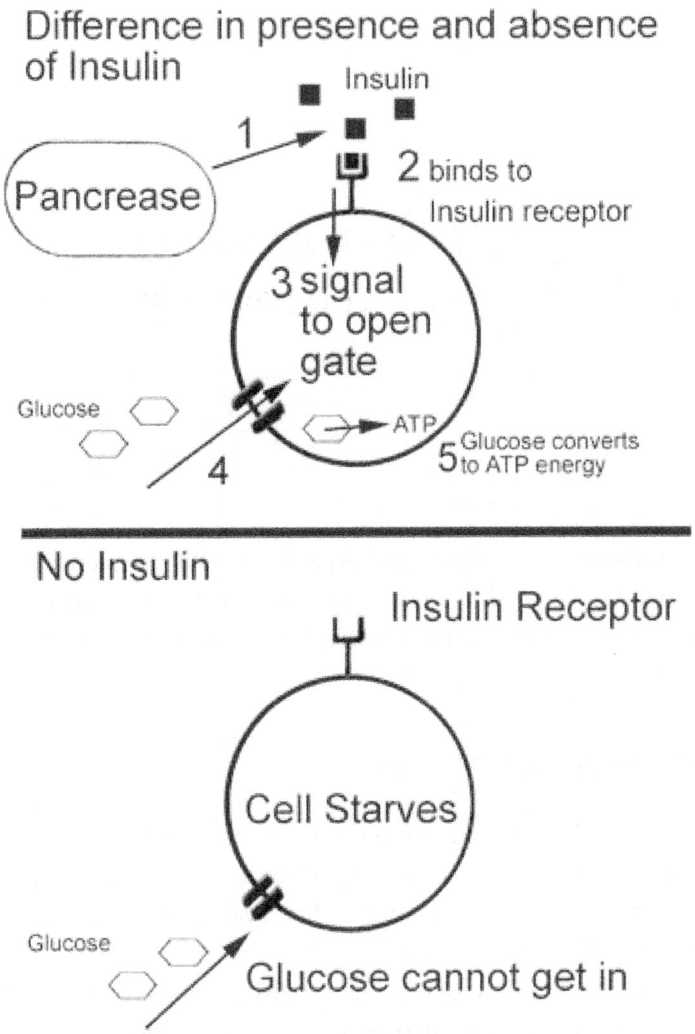
Difference in presence and absence of Insulin
Insulin
1
Pancrease
2 binds to Insulin receptor
3 signal to open gate
Glucose
4
ATP
5 Glucose converts to ATP energy
No Insulin
Insulin Receptor
Cell Starves
Glucose
Glucose cannot get in

Here are the different types of anti-diabetic drugs:

1. Oral Medications:

Sulfonylureas (SU): Examples include tolbutamide, glibenclamide, and nateglinide. These drugs stimulate insulin secretion from pancreatic beta cells.

2. Biguanides:

Metformin and buformin belong to this class. They reduce glucose production in the liver, inhibit intestinal glucose absorption, and enhance glucose uptake by skeletal muscles.

3. Insulin-Sensitizing Drugs:

Thiazolidinediones (TZDs), such as pioglitazone and rosiglitazone, improve insulin sensitivity in cells, particularly in obese individuals with insulin resistance.

4. α-Glucosidase Inhibitors:

Acarbose is an example of this class, which delays carbohydrate digestion in the intestines, leading to reduced postprandial blood sugar levels.

5. Aldose Reductase Inhibitors:

Epalrestat inhibits aldose reductase, an enzyme involved in the conversion of glucose to sorbitol. This helps prevent diabetic neuropathy and other complications associated with sorbitol accumulation.

6. Incretin Mimetics (GLP-1 Agonists)

GLP-1 Agonists: Revolutionizing Diabetes Management Incretin mimetics, such as Ozempic, are a breakthrough in the treatment of type 2 diabetes. Acting similarly to incretin hormones like glucagon-like peptide-1 (GLP-1), they bind to GLP-1 receptors, prompting glucose-dependent insulin release, effectively controlling hyperglycemia. Additionally, these agents curb appetite, suppress glucagon secretion, and delay gastric emptying, preventing rapid spikes in postprandial blood glucose levels. Ozempic, a long-acting injectable GLP-1 receptor agonist, offers a once-weekly treatment option for adults with type 2 diabetes. Clinical trials have even explored its potential for weight loss. After 30 weeks, patients on Ozempic exhibited significant weight reduction compared to the placebo group, with those on 0.5mg losing 2.6 kg more and those on 1mg shedding 3.5 kg more. Despite its efficacy in weight management, it's important to note that Ozempic is not currently FDA-approved for this purpose.

7. Injectable Insulin

For individuals with Type 1 diabetes, where the body no longer produces insulin, injecting insulin directly into the body is essential. Insulin acts as a signaling "flag" that prompts components involved in glucose metabolism to uptake glucose into the cells. Without this signaling mechanism, cells remain starved for energy, even in the presence of ample glucose in the bloodstream. Additionally, insulin signals the liver cells to regulate blood sugar levels by storing excess glucose as glycogen.

Managing diabetes requires a comprehensive approach involving medication, lifestyle modifications, and dietary changes. While oral medications are commonly used for Type 2 diabetes, insulin therapy is essential for individuals with Type 1 diabetes. Various types of insulin formulations are available, each with different onset and duration of action, to regulate blood sugar levels effectively.

In addition to conventional medications, natural remedies, and alternative therapies are also popular among individuals with diabetes. Herbs like cinnamon, bitter melon, and fenugreek, as well as supplements like chromium picolinate, have shown promise in improving blood sugar control and insulin sensitivity. However, it is essential to consult healthcare providers before incorporating these remedies into the treatment plan to ensure their safety and efficacy.

It is important for individuals with diabetes to work closely with their healthcare providers to determine the most appropriate medication regimen for their specific needs. By understanding how different medications work and their potential side effects, individuals can take control of their diabetes and lead a healthier, more fulfilling life.

Medication for Heart Failure

Heart failure, a condition where the heart is unable to pump enough blood to meet the body's needs, affects millions of people globally. Medications play a vital role in managing heart failure and enhancing patients' quality of life.

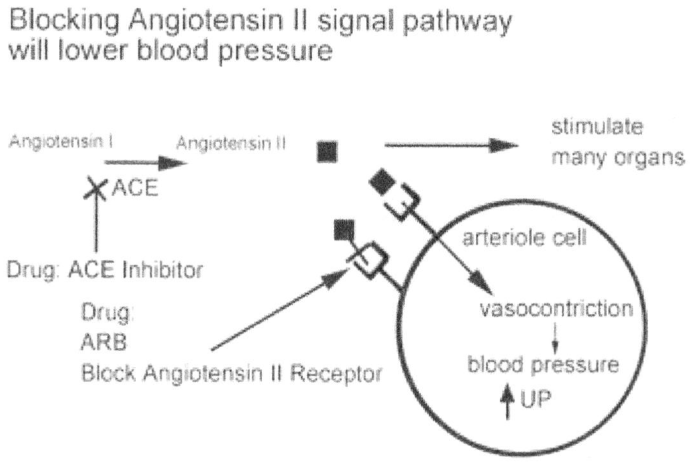

Several classes of medications are commonly used to treat heart failure, each targeting different aspects of the condition:

ACE Inhibitors

ACE inhibitors, like lisinopril and enalapril, work by inhibiting angiotensin-converting enzyme (ACE). This helps relax blood vessels, reduce the workload on the heart, and decrease blood pressure. ACE inhibitors are often the first choice for heart failure treatment, as they can alleviate symptoms and promote heart recovery. However, they may cause a persistent dry cough as a side effect due to increased bradykinin levels.

Angiotensin II Receptor Blockers (ARBs)

Similar to ACE inhibitors, ARBs such as losartan potassium also help relax blood vessels and lower blood pressure. However, they target angiotensin receptors instead of ACE enzymes. ARBs are an alternative option for patients who cannot tolerate ACE inhibitors.

Beta-1 Receptor Stimulants

Drugs like dopamine hydrochloride stimulate beta-1 receptors in the heart, leading to more forceful and complete contractions of the heart muscle cells. This helps improve cardiac output and alleviate symptoms of heart failure.

Phosphodiesterase III Inhibitors

Phosphodiesterase III inhibitors like milrinone enhance the effect of cyclic AMP (c-AMP) by increasing Ca2+-ATPase activity in cardiac muscle cells. This results in improved relaxation of the left ventricle of the heart, leading to increased heart contraction. These medications can be effective for patients with severe heart failure who do not respond adequately to other treatments.

Enhancing Cardiac Function

Cardiac glycosides, such as digoxin derived from digitalis plant leaves, exert crucial positive inotropic, neurohormonal, and electrophysiologic effects. These properties form the cornerstone of their application in managing two distinct clinical scenarios: heart failure stemming from systolic dysfunction and specific supraventricular tachyarrhythmias. Digoxin acts to strengthen the heart's contractions and promote a more regular rhythm, rendering it an invaluable tool in the treatment of heart failure. Moreover, it finds utility in addressing atrial fibrillation, a disorder characterized by irregular heartbeats originating in the upper chambers of the heart. For optimal early efficacy in managing tachyarrhythmias, digoxin necessitates loading doses, which may be administered intravenously or orally to achieve maximal benefits promptly.

It is crucial for patients with heart failure to adhere to their prescribed medication regimen. Skipping doses or abruptly stopping medication can exacerbate symptoms and lead to serious complications. Patients should also be vigilant about potential side effects and drug interactions, promptly reporting any concerns to their healthcare provider.

In addition to medication, lifestyle modifications such as maintaining a healthy diet, regular exercise, and smoking cessation can contribute to better heart failure management. By collaborating closely with healthcare providers and following a comprehensive treatment plan, individuals with heart failure can improve their prognosis and overall well-being.

A note on the use of beta-blockers in heart failure treatment:

Historically, there was concern that administering beta-blockers to patients with heart failure could exacerbate the condition by further weakening the heart. However, extensive research and clinical trials conducted since 2000 have provided compelling evidence that beta-blocker medications can be beneficial for many patients with heart failure. These drugs can help the heart by providing it with additional rest to facilitate recovery. It is essential, however, for patients to consult with their physician to determine the most appropriate beta-blocker medication for their heart failure treatment plan.

Medication for Hypertension (High Blood Pressure)

Hypertension, commonly known as high blood pressure, affects millions worldwide and is often termed the "silent killer" due to its typically asymptomatic nature but serious health implications if left untreated. Managing hypertension involves lifestyle modifications alongside medication, as it is a chronic condition requiring comprehensive care.

Here are the main types of anti-hypertension drugs:

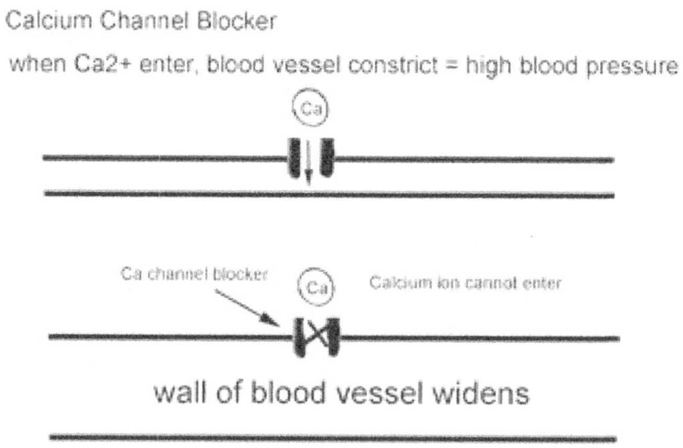

1. **Calcium Channel Blockers**
   These medications work by inhibiting calcium ions from entering smooth muscle cells in blood vessel walls, preventing their contraction and thus lowering blood pressure. Examples include amlodipine, aranidipine, and nifedipine.
2. **Angiotensin-Converting Enzyme (ACE) Inhibitors**
   ACE inhibitors, such as captopril and enalapril, block the conversion of angiotensin I to angiotensin II, thereby preventing blood vessel constriction and reducing blood pressure.
3. **Angiotensin II Receptor Blockers (ARBs)**
   ARBs, like losartan and candesartan, act on angiotensin II receptors, preventing their activation and consequent blood vessel constriction, effectively lowering blood pressure.
4. **Beta-blockers**

These medications, including propranolol and atenolol, target beta receptors primarily in the heart and kidneys, reducing heart rate and relaxing blood vessels to lower blood pressure. Beta-blockers are also beneficial for hypertension patients with arrhythmias.

5. **Diuretics**
   Diuretics, particularly thiazide-type drugs like hydrochlorothiazide and furosemide, help lower blood pressure by promoting the excretion of excess water and salt through urine, thereby reducing blood volume.
6. **Alpha-blockers**
   Alpha-blockers, such as prazosin and terazosin, act on alpha receptors in blood vessel walls to block their constriction, leading to vasodilation and decreased blood pressure.

While these medications effectively control blood pressure, there is currently no cure for hypertension, necessitating lifelong medication use. However, ongoing research suggests promising results for non-strenuous exercises like Tai Chi or Falun Gong as adjunctive therapies for hypertension management.

Patients must adhere to prescribed medication regimens and remain vigilant for potential side effects, working closely with healthcare providers to manage hypertension effectively and mitigate the risk of serious health complications.

Peptic Ulcer Treatment

Peptic ulcer, characterized by ulceration in the gastrointestinal (GI) tract, presents as a painful and potentially serious condition with risks of internal bleeding and complications. Helicobacter pylori bacterial infection and NSAID usage are common causes of peptic ulcers, necessitating effective treatment strategies.

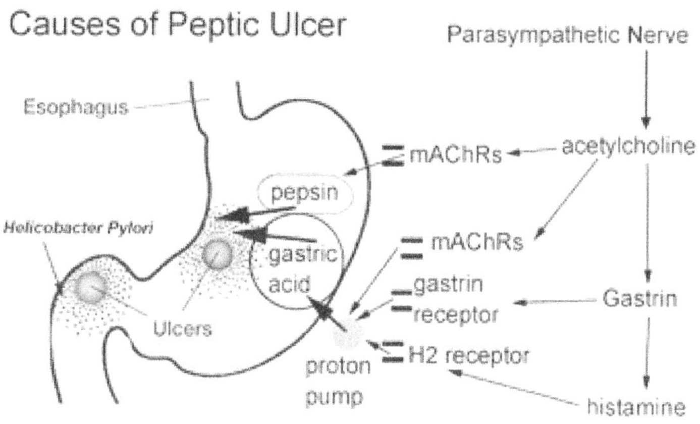

Here are the main treatments for peptic ulcer:

1. Antibiotics

Combating H. pylori infection is crucial in peptic ulcer treatment. Antibiotics like amoxicillin and clarithromycin are commonly prescribed alongside other medications to eradicate the bacteria and prevent ulcer recurrence.

2. Reducing Acidity Drugs

Lowering stomach acidity promotes ulcer healing. Various drugs achieve this through different mechanisms:

1. **H2 Blockers (Histamine H2 Antagonist):** Drugs like cimetidine and famotidine block histamine H2 receptors, reducing gastric acid production.
2. **Gastrin Inhibitors:** Proglumide inhibits gastrin activity, decreasing gastric acid secretion.
3. **Muscarinic Receptors (mAChRs) Inhibitors:** Copolamine butylbromide inhibits acetylcholine activity, reducing gastric acid secretion and alleviating pain.
4. **Proton Pump Inhibitors (PPIs):** Potent drugs like omeprazole inhibit gastric acid production at the final step, providing long-lasting acid suppression but potentially weakening the stomach's defense mechanisms.
5. **Antacids:** Neutralizing gastric acid with substances like dried aluminum hydroxide gel helps prevent further erosion of the ulcer and provides relief from symptoms.

3. Strengthen Stomach Drugs

Supporting stomach mucosa repair and protection is essential:

1. **Sucralfate:** Forms a protective barrier over the ulcer, shielding it from stomach acid.
2. **Aldioxa:** Promotes stomach cell wall repair.
3. **Teprenone:** Stimulates gastric mucosa production, enhancing the stomach's protective layer.
4. **Cetraxate Hydrochloride:** Promotes gastric mucosa production.

5. **Prostaglandin:** Synthetic prostaglandins like enprostil prevent and treat peptic ulcers by inhibiting gastric acid secretion and promoting cytoprotection of stomach mucosa. Treatment of peptic ulcers involves a multifaceted approach, often combining medication with lifestyle changes. Proton pump inhibitors (PPIs) and H2-receptor antagonists are commonly used drugs to reduce stomach acid production and promote ulcer healing. Avoiding NSAIDs, alcohol, and smoking, managing stress, and adopting a healthy diet are integral to ulcer management and prevention of complications.

By collaborating with healthcare providers and adhering to prescribed treatment regimens, individuals can effectively manage peptic ulcers and prevent recurrence, improving their quality of life and reducing the risk of complications.

Anti-osteoporosis Treatment

Osteoporosis, characterized by decreased bone density and increased fracture risk, is a prevalent condition, particularly among women and the elderly. Bone remodeling, a process involving both resorption by osteoclasts and formation by osteoblasts, maintains bone health. Osteoporosis arises when bone resorption exceeds formation, leading to bone weakening and increased fracture susceptibility.

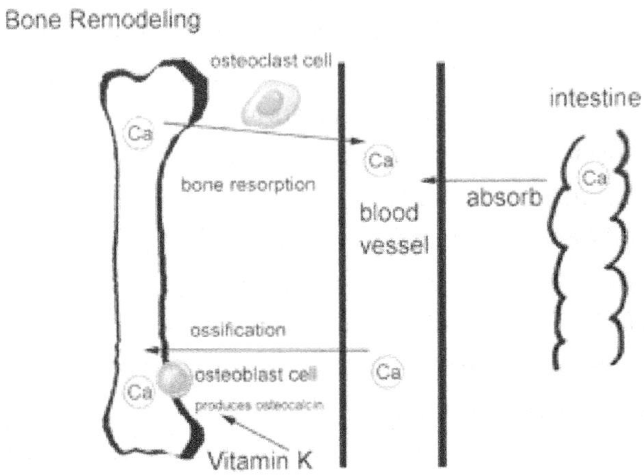

Here are the drugs used for osteoporosis treatment:

1. **Calcium Replenishers**

Calcium gluconate, calcium lactate, and calcium L-aspartate increase blood calcium levels, inhibiting osteoclast activity and promoting bone health.

2. **Active Form of Vitamin D (D3)**

Cholecalciferol, or vitamin D3, facilitates intestinal calcium absorption and elevates blood calcium levels, supporting bone strength.

3. **Estrogen Replacement**

Estrogen regulates osteoclast apoptosis, and its decline post-menopause contributes to osteoporosis. Estriol supplementation addresses estrogen deficiency.

4. **Selective Estrogen Modulators (SERMs)**

SERMs like raloxifene activate bone-building estrogen receptors without stimulating breast and uterine tissue, reducing osteoporosis risk without increasing cancer risk.

5. Antiresorptive Drugs

Elcatonin (ECT) alleviates postmenopausal osteoporosis pain by inhibiting bone resorption and promoting bone formation, sourced from eel and salmon.

6. Vitamin K

Vitamin K, crucial for bone formation, aids osteoblast activity and osteocalcin production, supporting bone density.

7. Bone Resorption Inhibitors

Synthetic bisphosphonates, such as etidronate disodium, inhibit bone breakdown, increasing bone density and reducing fracture risk.

8. Ipriflavone

Found in plants, ipriflavone inhibits bone resorption, promoting osteoblast activity and bone density, particularly in postmenopausal osteoporosis.

One of the primary treatments for osteoporosis is bisphosphonates, which slow bone tissue breakdown, increasing bone density and fracture resistance. Additionally, hormone replacement therapy and selective estrogen receptor modulators can increase bone formation or reduce bone resorption.

Lifestyle modifications, including weight-bearing exercise and a diet rich in calcium and vitamin D, complement medication therapy for osteoporosis. Natural supplements like calcium, magnesium, and vitamin K may also support bone health, but consultation with a healthcare provider is essential to ensure compatibility with existing treatments.

In conclusion, osteoporosis treatment involves a multifaceted approach integrating medication, lifestyle adjustments, and potentially natural supplements. Collaborating with healthcare providers enables individuals to tailor treatment plans to their specific needs and goals, optimizing osteoporosis management and fracture prevention.

Treatments for Thyroid Disease

The thyroid gland in the neck plays a vital role in controlling and regulating hormone levels in the blood and the body's metabolism. It secretes thyroid hormones T3 and T4, with T3 directly utilized by cells for protein production. T4, upon entering cells, undergoes conversion into T3. Certain thyroid diseases stem from autoimmune disorders, making it challenging to treat the underlying cause. Consequently, many drugs focus on regulating normal thyroid function rather than addressing autoimmune-induced diseases directly. Thyroid disease, affecting millions globally, disrupts hormone regulation and metabolism, leading to varied symptoms like fatigue, weight changes, and mood swings. While some conditions arise from autoimmune disorders, treatment focuses on regulating thyroid function rather than curing autoimmune causes.

Here are the major drugs used for thyroid disease treatment:

1. Hormone Replacement Therapy for Hypothyroidism

- **Desiccated Thyroid:** A natural substance containing both T3 and T4, derived from pig glands, used to treat hypothyroidism. However, some patients may be allergic to it due to its source variability.
- **Synthetic T4 (Levothyroxine):** A synthetic form of T4 that can be readily converted into T3 by cells, used to replace deficient thyroid hormones.

- **Synthetic T3 (Liothyronine):** Directly increases metabolic rate and promotes protein synthesis, aiding in hypothyroidism treatment.

2. **Treatment for Hyperthyroidism or Overactive Thyroid:**

   1. **Thyroperoxidase Inhibitor (Thiamazole):** This drug inhibits the enzyme thyroperoxidase, which is essential for thyroid hormone synthesis, thus reducing hormone concentration.
   2. **Iodine:** Excessive intake can inhibit thyroid hormone production, often used alongside anti-thyroid drugs before surgery to lower hormone levels.
   3. **Other Treatments for Thyroid Disease:**

- **Surgery:** Removal of part or all of the thyroid gland may be necessary to address nodules or tumors causing dysfunction.
- **Radioactive Iodine Therapy:** Targets and destroys thyroid tissue using a radioactive form of iodine.
- **Alternative Treatments:** Dietary changes, supplements like selenium or zinc, and lifestyle modifications can complement traditional treatments, offering relief from symptoms and supporting thyroid health.

Ultimately, effective thyroid disease management requires collaboration with healthcare providers to tailor treatment plans to individual needs. Exploring various treatment options allows individuals to find relief from symptoms and improve overall health and well-being.

Medication for Angina Pectoris

Sufficient oxygen supply and nutrients are vital for the proper functioning of heart cells, as the heart muscles constantly work to maintain bodily functions. Coronary arteries are responsible for supplying blood to the heart. Any issues with these arteries can impair heart function and potentially lead to fatal consequences. Angina pectoris occurs when there is inadequate oxygen supply to the heart muscle, often resulting in severe chest pain or discomfort. This condition, commonly associated with underlying heart conditions such as coronary artery disease, necessitates effective management through medications to improve individuals' quality of life.

To address angina pectoris effectively, medications target two primary objectives: increasing oxygen supply to coronary arteries and reducing the heart's workload. Here are the key drug classes used in treating angina pectoris:

1. **Nitrates:** An exemplary drug in this category is nitroglycerin. Nitroglycerin has been recognized for its utility since its historical application in explosives during the 1800s. However, it also serves as a medication for treating angina by effectively dilating blood vessels through the relaxation of smooth muscle cells in the vessel walls. This action enhances the capacity of coronary arteries to deliver oxygen while simultaneously reducing the volume of blood in the heart. By facilitating increased oxygen supply to the heart and reducing its workload, nitroglycerin plays a crucial role in managing angina. Mechanistically, nitroglycerin promotes the production of nitric oxide in the body, which leads to the conversion of cyclic guanosine

triphosphates (GTP) to cyclic guanosine monophosphate (c-GMP). Elevated levels of c-GMP trigger the relaxation of heart muscle cells by reducing the concentration of calcium ions (Ca2+) within the cells, resulting in the widening of arteries.

2. **Calcium Channel Blockers:** These drugs lower blood pressure by obstructing calcium ions' entry into calcium channels, subsequently reducing the heart's workload. Additionally, they stabilize coronary artery spasms, preventing angina recurrence. Examples include nitrendipine, benidipine, nisoldipine, and verapamil.
3. **Beta-blockers:** By slowing the heart rate and decreasing blood pressure, beta-blockers alleviate the heart's oxygen demand, thereby preventing angina episodes and enhancing exercise tolerance. Common examples are atenolol, carvedilol, and labetalol.
4. **Coronary Arterial Vasodilators:** These vasodilators effectively prevent angina recurrence by widening the blood vessels of the heart arteries. For instance, Nicorandil operates by facilitating nitric oxide production, which then interacts with guanylate cyclase, the enzyme responsible for synthesizing c-GMP. This process leads to a rapid increase in the concentration of c-GMP, prompting the flow of calcium ions and resulting in the dilation of both arterial (blood flowing into the heart) and venous (blood flowing out from the heart) vessels. Other examples of vasodilators include dipyridamole and dilazep hydrochloride. Other examples include dipyridamole and dilazep hydrochloride.

Individuals with angina pectoris should collaborate closely with their healthcare providers to devise a suitable medication regimen tailored to their needs. Adhering to prescribed dosages and instructions ensures optimal efficacy and minimizes potential side effects.

Moreover, alongside medication, lifestyle modifications such as regular exercise, a balanced diet, stress management, and smoking cessation are integral in managing angina pectoris effectively. By adopting a comprehensive approach to treatment, individuals with angina pectoris can enhance their quality of life and reduce the risk of associated complications.

Anti-thrombotic Drugs

Thrombosis, the formation of blood clots within blood vessels, poses significant health risks, especially when occurring in critical areas like the brain or heart. Anti-thrombotic drugs play a crucial role in modern medicine, aiming to prevent clot formation and mitigate associated complications.

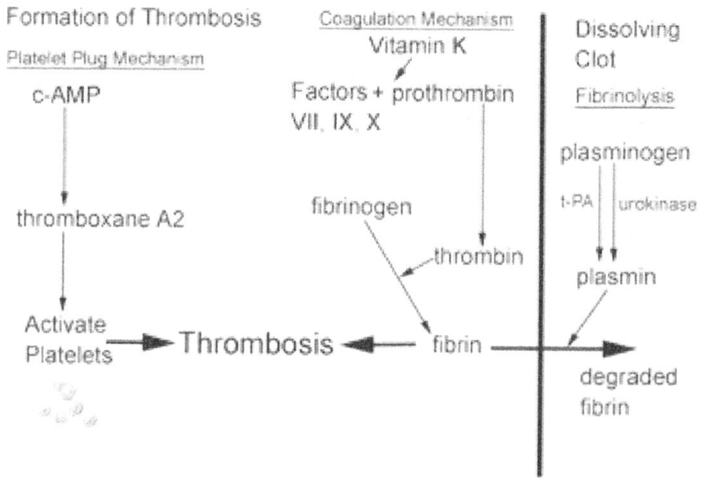

Here's a breakdown of the different types of anti-thrombotic drugs:

Platelet Plug Mechanism Inhibitors:

1. Aspirin (acetylsalicylic acid):

Aspirin inhibits the synthesis of thromboxane A2, a substance crucial for blood clot formation, by blocking prostaglandin production. However, proper dosage is essential as excessive aspirin can reverse its effects.

2. Ozagrel Sodium:

This medication inhibits thromboxane A2 synthesis and conversion, effectively preventing platelet aggregation, especially in smaller blood vessels, making it beneficial for cerebral thrombosis.

3. Ticlopidine:

Ticlopidine alters platelet membranes, hindering their aggregation with fibrinogens. It also increases c-AMP concentration, further inhibiting thromboxane A2 production.

4. Sarpogrelate hydrochloride:

Acting as a 5-HT2 receptor antagonist, this drug prevents platelet aggregation by inhibiting serotonin's effect on platelets.

Coagulation Mechanism Inhibitors:

1. Heparin Sodium:

Heparin, a natural anticoagulant, interferes with thrombin's functionality, impeding fibrin formation from fibrinogen.

2. Warfarin:

By antagonizing vitamin K, essential for synthesizing coagulation factors, Warfarin effectively inhibits coagulation.

Fibrin Dissolvers:

1. Urokinase:

Naturally occurring, urokinase catalyzes the conversion of plasminogen to plasmin, initiating the dissolution of blood clots. It's usually administered locally to avoid internal bleeding.

2. Tissue Plasminogen Activator (t-PA):

These drugs, like alteplase and others, are utilized in conditions like heart attacks or strokes to dissolve blood clots effectively.

It's essential for individuals taking anti-thrombotic drugs to adhere to prescribed dosages and report any adverse effects promptly. Besides traditional medications, natural supplements like fish oil and garlic also offer alternatives for individuals unable to tolerate conventional anti-thrombotic drugs. Understanding how these medications function empowers individuals to manage their risk of thrombosis effectively and maintain their well-being.

Medications for Migraine

Migraine, characterized by abnormal constriction and dilation of blood vessels in the head region, remains a condition with an unknown precise cause. Two prevailing theories, the Platelet Theory and the Trigeminal Nerve Theory, guide the development of medications aimed at addressing migraine symptoms.

Theories Explaining Migraine Causes:

1. Platelet Theory:

Stress, sensory stimuli, and sleep disturbances can activate platelet mechanisms, leading to abnormal serum levels and vasodilation, triggering nerve system abnormalities.

2. Trigeminal Nerve Theory:

Repetitive pains and headaches are believed to originate in or be related to the Trigeminal Nerve.

Drugs for Acute Migraine Attack:

1. Ergotamine:

Mechanism: Acts as a 5-HT receptor agonist, causing vasoconstriction due to its structural similarity to neurotransmitters like serotonin. Example: Dihydroergotamine mesilate.

2. NSAIDs:

Mechanism: Inhibits prostaglandin synthesis by COX-2, reducing pain levels. Example: Aspirin.

3. Sumatriptan:

Mechanism: Acts as a 5-HT 1D agonist, constricting blood vessels back to normal. Also inhibits Calcitonin gene-related peptide (CGRP) release from Trigeminal ganglion, reducing pain.

Drugs for Migraine Prevention:

1. Calcium Channel Blockers:

Mechanism: Used to lower blood pressure, but also helpful in widening blood vessels to prevent migraines. Example: Lomerizine hydrochloride. Not for use during acute migraine attacks.

2. Beta-blockers:

Mechanism: Used to lower blood pressure, and relax blood vessels, preventing migraines. Example: Propranolol.

3. Antidepressant Drugs:

Example: Amitriptyline.

Mechanism: Increases levels of serotonin and norepinephrine in the brain. Dosage varies among patients. Caution is needed when used concurrently with other drugs or herbal supplements like St. John's wort to avoid adverse interactions.

Understanding these mechanisms and medications is crucial for effectively managing migraine symptoms and improving the quality of life for individuals affected by this condition.

4

Chapter 4: Drugs that you too can understand if you really want to know. Just take a little bit more time

Treatment for Epilepsy

Epilepsy is a neurological disorder characterized by recurrent seizures. These seizures can vary in intensity and duration, often causing disruptions in a person's daily life. Fortunately, there are several treatment options available for individuals with epilepsy that can help manage their symptoms and improve their quality of life. Our brain is a complex network of neurons that communicate via electrical signals. However, when there's abnormal and excessive neuronal activity, it can lead to seizures—a hallmark of epilepsy. Epilepsy, a chronic neurological disorder, currently has no cure. Convulsions, marked by uncontrolled shaking or muscle contractions, are common during seizures. Anticonvulsant drugs aim to suppress this excessive neuronal firing.

Medication is a primary treatment for epilepsy. Antiepileptic drugs (AEDs) help reduce the frequency and severity of seizures by stabilizing electrical activity in the brain. Adherence to prescribed medication and regular follow-ups with healthcare providers are essential.

Beyond medication, alternative therapies like dietary changes (e.g., ketogenic diet), acupuncture, or biofeedback may benefit some individuals.

For severe or drug-resistant epilepsy cases, surgery might be considered to remove seizure-originating brain areas, reducing future seizure risks.

Treatment for epilepsy is highly individualized and may involve a combination of approaches. Active collaboration between individuals with epilepsy and healthcare providers is crucial to develop effective treatment plans.

Below are medications commonly used to control epilepsy:

1. Sodium Valproate: Blocks signal transmission in voltage-gated sodium and calcium channels, increasing gamma-aminobutyric acid (GABA) levels—a neurotransmitter that inhibits central nervous system activity.
2. Carbamazepine: Stabilizes sodium channel inactivation, reducing excessive neuronal firing.
3. Phenytoin: Stabilizes sodium channel inactivation, particularly useful for chronic muscle spasms with pain.
4. Ethosuximide: Blocks T-type calcium channels involved in signal transmission timing.
5. Phenobarbital: Enhances GABA activity, blocks sodium channels, and acts as a sedative and hypnotic.
6. Primidone: Inhibits action potentials generated by voltage-gated sodium channels, particularly for secondarily gener-

alized seizures.

7. Clonazepam: Activates GABA receptors, inhibiting central nervous system synaptic transmission.
8. Gabapentin: Structurally similar to GABA, may relieve pain by blocking T-type calcium channels and increasing GABA levels.

Antibiotics

Antibiotics are potent medications used to combat bacterial infections by either killing bacteria or halting their reproduction. While they can be life-saving, it's crucial to use them responsibly to prevent antibiotic resistance.

Bacterial infections occur when foreign substances invade the body, leading to their proliferation. Microorganisms like bacteria, fungi, or viruses can replicate within the body. Unlike bacteria, prions—primarily protein-based—don't self-replicate. Antibiotics target bacteria, while antivirals and antifungals combat viruses and fungi, respectively.

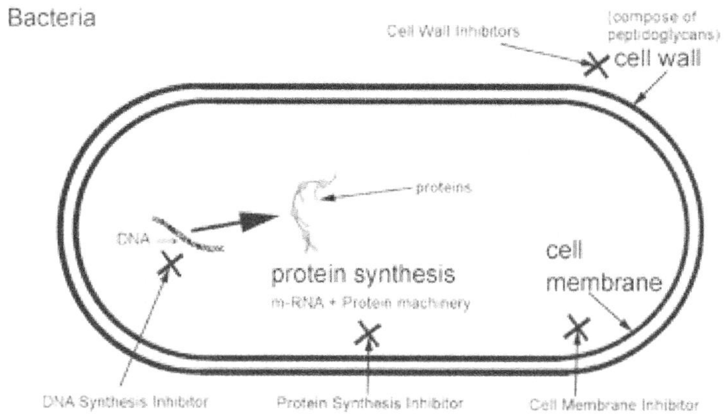

Antibiotics primarily inhibit bacterial growth, tackling various mechanisms:

1. **Beta-lactam Antibiotics** – Cell Wall Inhibitors: Penicillins and cephems disrupt bacterial cell walls, weakening them and causing rupture. These disrupt the bacterial cell wall because their structure resembles a component of the cell wall called peptidoglycan. However, unlike natural peptidoglycans, these drugs do not form cross-links with other peptidoglycans to create the mesh-like layer. Consequently, the cell wall weakens, leading to its rupture when the bacteria are unable to maintain functional pressure.
2. **Cell Membrane Inhibitors:** Polymyxin B binds to bacterial cell membranes, making them permeable and leading to cell death.
3. **Protein Synthesis Inhibitors:** Drugs like tetracycline hinder bacterial protein synthesis by blocking ribosome

binding sites. As you may be aware, proteins are synthesized in a step-by-step process resembling an assembly line. This process begins with the copying of instructions from DNA onto messenger RNA (mRNA). The mRNA then carries these instructions to the ribosome, where protein synthesis takes place. Tetracycline, an example of these drugs, can permanently inhibit the binding site of the ribosome, which is the protein machinery responsible for assembling proteins.

4. **DNA Synthesis Inhibitors:** Quinolones prevent bacterial DNA unwinding, crucial for transcription, akin to opening a book to read. Just as you need to open a book to read a specific page, DNA must unwind before messenger RNA (mRNA) can be produced from it. Quinolones possess the ability to impede this unwinding process in DNA, similar to preventing the opening of a book to a particular page.
5. **Beta-lactamase Inhibitors:** Drugs like clavulanic acid assist antibiotics by inhibiting bacterial beta-lactamase, restoring antibiotic efficacy. This class of drugs isn't technically an antibiotic, but it aids antibiotics in eliminating bacteria. Certain bacteria develop resistance to beta-lactam antibiotics by producing an enzyme called beta-lactamase (penicillinase), which breaks down the beta-lactam ring, rendering these drugs ineffective. However, a breakthrough was made with the use of beta-lactamase inhibitors like clavulanic acid, which enhance the effectiveness of beta-lactam antibiotics by neutralizing the bacterial enzyme.
6. **Mupirocin:** Topical antibiotic inhibiting RNA synthesis, used for treating MRSA infections. This antibiotic is also effective against methicillin-resistant Staphylococcus

aureus (MRSA), a bacteria commonly found on the skin. However, it's typically used as a topical treatment. It works by inhibiting RNA synthesis, preventing the production of bacterial proteins. Nonetheless, there have been studies indicating that Staphylococcus bacteria may develop resistance to mupirocin.

7. **Vancomycin:** Reserved as a last resort for MRSA infections, it disrupts cell wall synthesis. MRSA bacteria are typically resistant to numerous antibiotics. Vancomycin is reserved as a "last resort" treatment for MRSA infections, used only when other antibiotics have failed. It functions by inhibiting cell wall synthesis, incorporating itself into the peptidoglycan cross-linked matrix. However, there have been instances of bacteria developing resistance to vancomycin.
8. **Last Line of Defense:** Linezolid and daptomycin serve as alternatives when vancomycin fails, disrupting bacterial protein synthesis and various metabolic processes. As vancomycin's effectiveness diminishes, both linezolid and daptomycin have emerged as alternatives. Linezolid, introduced in 2009 as a newer synthetic antibiotic, inhibits bacterial protein synthesis, disrupting growth. Meanwhile, daptomycin disrupts multiple bacterial metabolic processes, including cell membrane function, DNA and RNA, and protein synthesis. This ongoing quest for new antibiotics reflects the perpetual battle between humans and bacteria.

Awareness of antibiotic side effects is crucial, including upset stomach, diarrhea, and allergic reactions. Adhering to prescribed dosages and treatment durations is vital to prevent antibiotic resistance.

Nurses and healthcare workers educate patients on antibiotic use, monitor adverse reactions, and report concerns. Alternative medicine practitioners advocate for natural remedies like probiotics and herbal supplements to support the immune system. Patients must consult healthcare providers before taking antibiotics, providing thorough medical histories and allergy information.

In conclusion, antibiotics are indispensable for bacterial infections but must be used cautiously to prevent resistance and side effects. Collaboration among healthcare providers, patients, and alternative medicine practitioners ensures responsible antibiotic use for optimal patient outcomes.

Treatment for Parkinson's disease

Parkinson's disease (PD) results from a deficiency in dopamine production in the brain, although its exact cause remains elusive. This deficiency stems from decreased activity of dopaminergic cells in the brain's substantia nigra. Dopamine, a neurotransmitter and neurohormone, serves various functions in the central nervous system.

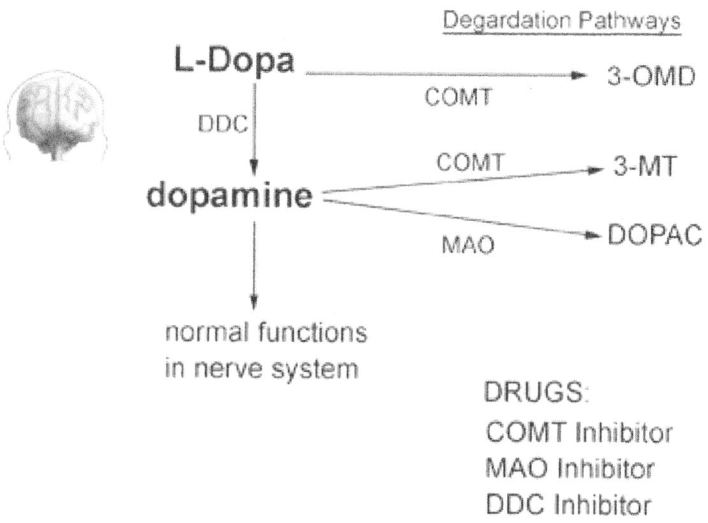

Medications for Parkinson's disease primarily aim to boost dopamine levels. Here's a breakdown of these drugs:

1. **L-Dopa (Levodopa):** Since dopamine cannot effectively cross the blood-brain barrier, its precursor, L-Dopa, is administered. Once in the brain, L-Dopa converts into dopamine, replenishing depleted stores.
2. **Amantadine:** While its exact mechanism remains unclear, amantadine is thought to enhance dopamine production and reabsorption. It's typically used in the early stages of the disease.
3. **Dopamine Agonists:** Drugs like pramipexole, ropinirole, and cabergoline bind to dopamine receptors, mimicking dopamine's actions.
4. **Acetylcholine Inhibitors:** Trihexyphenidyl hydrochloride

is an example of drugs that rebalance acetylcholine and dopamine levels, addressing symptoms like tremors and stiffness.

5. **Adrenaline Precursors:** Droxidopa maintains dopamine levels by preventing degradation. It converts into norepinephrine and epinephrine, hormones that play crucial roles in neurotransmitter concentration.
6. **Monoamine Oxidase B Inhibitors (MAOI-Bs)**: Selegiline and rasagiline inhibit dopamine breakdown, increasing its availability.
7. **COMT Inhibitors:** Entacapone and tolcapone prevent dopamine breakdown. Additionally, carbidopa and benserazide inhibit DDC to preserve L-Dopa levels.

Parkinson's disease treatment often involves a combination of medications, lifestyle adjustments, and, in some cases, surgical interventions. Dopamine agonists and levodopa-carbidopa combinations are commonly used to manage symptoms.

Lifestyle changes such as exercise and therapy can complement medication. For advanced cases, deep brain stimulation (DBS) surgery may be considered to regulate abnormal brain activity associated with Parkinson's disease.

Overall, treatment for Parkinson's disease is individualized based on the patient's symptoms, age, overall health, and other factors. It is important for patients to work closely with their healthcare providers to develop a comprehensive treatment plan that addresses their unique needs and goals.

Treatment for Arthritis

Arthritis, a prevalent condition affecting millions globally, manifests with joint pain, swelling, and stiffness. While its exact cause remains elusive, it's believed to be an autoimmune disease wherein the immune system targets its own tissues, leading to lifelong symptoms of pain and inflammation. Though no cure exists for Rheumatoid Arthritis (RA), two main treatment approaches aim to alleviate pain and prevent irreversible damage.

1. **NSAIDs:** Nonsteroidal anti-inflammatory drugs like diclofenac sodium alleviate RA pain by blocking the enzyme COX, which produces prostaglandins, thereby reducing pain and inflammation.
2. **Steroidal Anti-inflammatory Drugs:** Glucocorticoids such as prednisolone reduce inflammation by binding cortisol receptors, stimulating the production of anti-inflammatory proteins. Additionally, they suppress the immune system by reducing various immune cell populations.
3. **Antirheumatic Drugs:** Gold-based medications like sodium aurothiomalate or Gold Salt effectively reduce inflammation and provide longer-term relief.
4. **Disease Modifying Anti-Rheumatic Drugs (DMARDs):** Methotrexate, an example of DMARDs, is crucial, especially in early-stage RA, as it helps reduce damage to bone, cartilage, and joints. Methotrexate inhibits DNA synthesis and T-cell activity, delaying joint damage and preventing further inflammation. Methotrexate, an example of DMARDs, delays structural joint damage. Acting as an in-

hibitor of DNA synthesis, it blocks the enzyme responsible for converting folic acid into the DNA component pyrimidine. Additionally, methotrexate may inhibit T cells from releasing interleukins, thereby preventing neutrophils from causing further tissue damage and inflammation. However, it's important to note that methotrexate can be toxic if not used carefully.

Nonsteroidal anti-inflammatory drugs (NSAIDs) are commonly used to manage arthritis symptoms by reducing pain and inflammation. Corticosteroids offer fast relief when injected into affected joints but should be used cautiously due to potential side effects.

In addition to medications, physical therapy and exercise improve joint flexibility and strength. Some individuals find relief through natural remedies like turmeric, ginger, and fish oil supplements, which have anti-inflammatory properties.

Collaboration with healthcare providers is essential to tailor treatment plans to individual needs and goals. By combining medication, physical therapy, and lifestyle changes, individuals can effectively manage arthritis symptoms and enhance their overall quality of life.

In conclusion, a range of treatment options exists for arthritis, from medications to natural remedies and lifestyle adjustments. With guidance from healthcare providers, individuals can find relief from arthritis pain and improve their quality of life.

Medication for Bronchitis

Bronchitis, a respiratory condition marked by inflammation of the bronchial tubes, often presents with symptoms like coughing, wheezing, and breathing difficulties. While rest and home remedies suffice for most cases, medication may be necessary for others to alleviate symptoms and expedite recovery. The focus of bronchitis treatment has shifted towards reducing inflammation rather than solely targeting airway obstruction. Below are the treatments available for bronchitis.

1. **Beta-adrenergic Receptor Stimulant**

For acute bronchitis triggered by bacterial infections, antibiotics may be prescribed. Completing the full antibiotic course is vital to prevent antibiotic resistance and recurring infections. This drug is classified as a bronchodilator, working to elevate the level of cyclic AMP (cAMP), thereby widening the airways in the lungs. As cAMP levels rise, it influences dendritic cells in the immune system to decrease mucus secretion and reduce inflammation in lung tissue. In essence, it relaxes smooth muscle, facilitating the opening of respiratory airways. Examples of such drugs include beclometasone dipropionate and budesonide.

2. **Theophylline**

Bronchodilators, such as beta-adrenergic receptor stimulants, are often used to relax airway muscles, reducing inflammation and mucus secretion. Theophylline, another bronchodilator, aids in muscle relaxation and boasts anti-inflammatory properties. Theophylline is naturally present in tea, which is why the names of drugs containing it in many Asian countries include the word "tea." However, the concentration of theophylline in tea is insufficient to reach therapeutic levels.

Nowadays, many inhalers have replaced theophylline with anti-inflammatory steroids due to its numerous side effects and high likelihood of interacting with other drugs.

3. Steroidal Anti-inflammatory Drugs

Steroidal anti-inflammatory drugs like beclometasone dipropionate and budesonide effectively reduce inflammation and swelling by bolstering the production of anti-inflammatory proteins. These drugs, often administered via inhalers, target respiratory airways without penetrating the body, minimizing systemic side effects.

4. Anticholinergic Agents

Anticholinergic agents, like ipratropium, block muscarinic cholinergic receptors, reducing airway smooth muscle constriction. Antihistamines, such as sodium cromoglicate, stabilize mast cells, inhibiting histamine release and allergic reactions. It inhibits muscarinic cholinergic receptors, leading to a reduction in the level of c-GMP, ultimately indirectly preventing constriction in the smooth muscle of the airways.

5. Anti-allergic Agents (Antihistamine)

Anti-allergic agents come in various forms, including mast cell stabilizers like sodium cromoglicate, leukotriene antagonists like montelukast, and thromboxane receptor antagonists like seratrodast. Platelet-activating factor inhibitors like epinastine and cytokine inhibitors like suplatast tosilate also mitigate airway inflammation.

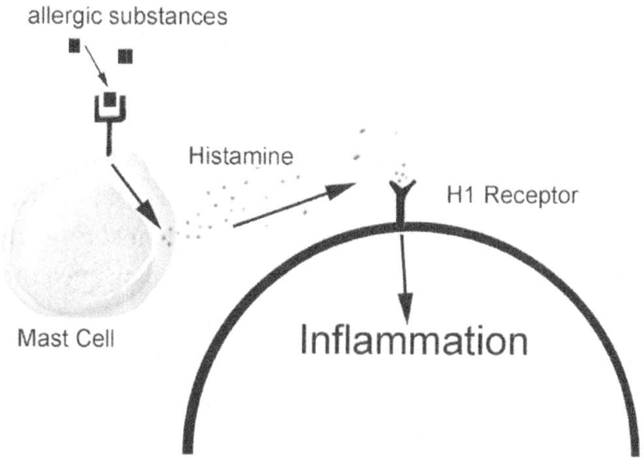

1. **Mast Cell Stabilizers (Anti-histamines)**

Medications like sodium cromoglicate work by inhibiting the release of histamine from mast cells, thereby reducing allergic reactions.

2. **Leukotriene Antagonists (Anti-Leukotrienes)**

These drugs, such as montelukast, prevent inflammation in conditions like asthma and bronchitis by blocking the production of leukotrienes, which are molecules that induce inflammatory effects.

3. **Thromboxane Receptor Antagonists**

These medications target the thromboxane receptor to treat chronic bronchitis. While the exact mechanism is not fully understood, research suggests that by deactivating the thromboxane receptor, drugs like seratrodast may suppress chronic coughing.

4. **Platelet-Activating Factor Inhibitors (Anti-PAF)**

Platelet-activating factors, produced in various organs including the lungs, can exacerbate airway inflammation. Drugs like epinastine inhibit these factors, reducing airway inflammation and improving symptoms of bronchitis.

5. Cytokine Inhibitors

This newer class of anti-allergic agents, such as suplatast tosilate, act by inhibiting the production of interleukin (IL) from T-cell helpers (Th-2 cells). Although not FDA-approved, suplatast tosilate has been available in Japan since 1995 and shows promise in reducing allergic reactions.

Individuals with bronchitis should collaborate closely with healthcare providers to devise suitable medication regimens. Adherence to prescribed instructions, including proper inhaler use and vigilant monitoring for side effects, is crucial. Additionally, staying hydrated, getting ample rest, and avoiding irritants like cigarette smoke and air pollution can complement medication efforts, enhancing symptom relief and overall quality of life.

Sleep Aid and Anti-anxiety

In today's fast-paced world, stress and anxiety are prevalent issues that many individuals encounter regularly, often leading to difficulties with sleep. Fortunately, there exists a range of sleep aids and anti-anxiety medications designed to alleviate these symptoms and foster a more restful night's sleep.

While most cases of insomnia and excessive anxiety stem from various stressors, these medications can provide valuable support. They aim to regulate signals within the nervous system. However, it's essential to address the underlying reasons for these conditions to achieve long-term relief.

Here are the medications for anti-anxiety:

1. Benzodiazepines (Benzo)

This class of drugs shares a common structure comprising a benzene ring and a diazepine. When individuals experience anxiety or excitement, various neurons become stimulated. Benzodiazepines work by inhibiting elements such as adrenaline, dopamine, and serotonin, thereby alleviating symptoms of anxiety and insomnia. For instance, chlordiazepoxide acts on the GABA (inhibitory neurotransmitter) subreceptor within the benzodiazepine system, leading to increased GABA levels that inhibit dopamine, adrenaline, and serotonin-related pathways.

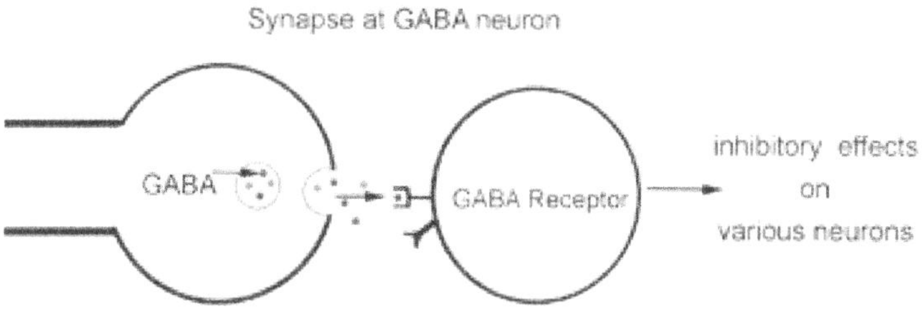

2. Tricyclic Antidepressants

Characterized by their three-ring structure, these drugs, such as imipramine, act similarly to benzodiazepines by targeting the benzodiazepine subreceptor of the GABA system.

3. 5-HT1A Receptor Partial Agonists

Tandospirone is an example of this type of drug, acting on the 5-HT1A receptor of serotonin to mediate inhibitory neurotransmission. Although it has a shorter half-life, it tends to have fewer side effects.

4. Benzodiazepines as Sleep Aids

Various benzodiazepines are used to treat insomnia, categorized by their duration of action. Examples include triazolam and brotizolam for fast-acting but short-term effects, and flurazepam and lorazepam for medium-term effects. However, longer-acting benzodiazepines like nitrazepam and diazepam are not recommended due to their persistence into the next day.

In addition to pharmaceutical options, natural remedies like melatonin and valerian root can aid sleep by promoting relaxation and reducing the time it takes to fall asleep. These alternatives offer a holistic approach to improving sleep quality but should be used under the guidance of a healthcare provider.

For individuals with severe anxiety, prescription medications such as benzodiazepines (e.g., Xanax, Valium) or selective serotonin reuptake inhibitors (SSRIs) like Prozac and Zoloft may be necessary. These medications regulate neurotransmitters to reduce anxiety and induce feelings of calmness.

It's essential to acknowledge that while these medications can effectively address sleep issues and anxiety, they carry potential side effects and risks. Close collaboration with a healthcare provider is crucial to develop an appropriate treatment plan and monitor for adverse reactions.

In summary, sleep aids and anti-anxiety medications serve as valuable tools in managing stress and promoting better sleep. By taking proactive steps towards mental health, individuals can enhance their overall well-being and quality of life.

Treatments for Depression

Depression, a widespread mental health disorder affecting millions globally, manifests through symptoms like difficulty concentrating, fatigue, and feelings of hopelessness. Its causes are intricate, often stemming from both individual predispositions and environmental factors.

The primary pharmacological approach to depression involves antidepressants, although they do not cure the condition but help manage its symptoms. These drugs target biochemical imbalances within synaptic transmissions, where neurotransmitter levels may be insufficient or receptor abundance excessive. Various antidepressant classes address these mechanisms:

1. Tricyclic Antidepressants (TCAs)

With a tricyclic ring structure, TCAs like imipramine elevate monoamine levels, including serotonin, norepinephrine, and dopamine.

2. Tetracyclic Antidepressants (TeCAs)

Having four-ring structures, TeCAs, akin to TCAs, inhibit monoamine reuptake, thereby boosting monoamine concentrations.

3. Selective Serotonin Reuptake Inhibitors (SSRIs)

SSRIs primarily target serotonin reuptake, offering fewer anticholinergic side effects compared to TCAs and TeCAs. Common examples include fluvoxamine, paroxetine (Paxil), citalopram, fluoxetin (Prozac), dapoxetine, escitalopram, sertraline (Zoloft), and zimelidine.

4. Serotonin-Norepinephrine Reuptake Inhibitors (SNRIs)

Unlike SSRIs, SNRIs like venlafaxine inhibit both serotonin and norepinephrine reuptake, demonstrating higher efficacy and fewer side effects. Unlike SSRIs, these medications additionally inhibit the reuptake of both norepinephrine and serotonin. This class of drugs, newer than SSRIs, has shown superior antidepressant efficacy and fewer side effects compared to TCAs and TeCAs. Examples include desvenlafaxine, venlafaxine, tramadol, duloxetine, and bicifadine.

5. Monoamine Oxidase Inhibitors (MAOIs)

Nonselective MAOIs such as phenelzine inhibit both MAO-alpha and MAO-beta, preventing monoamine degradation and increasing neurotransmitter availability. However, their use requires dietary restrictions due to potential interactions with tyramine-containing foods, such as cheese, avocados, and soy products, since it will dramatically increase blood pressure when tyramine interacts with MAOIs.

Antidepressants often necessitate several weeks to achieve therapeutic effects, and discontinuation should be gradual to avoid withdrawal symptoms.

Beyond medication, therapy plays a pivotal role in depression management. Cognitive-behavioral therapy (CBT) is widely employed, focusing on altering negative thought patterns and behaviors contributing to depressive symptoms. Alternative treatments like acupuncture, yoga, and meditation offer holistic approaches, emphasizing relaxation and stress reduction.

It's crucial for individuals with depression to collaborate with healthcare providers to tailor treatment plans to their needs. Through exploration and patience, individuals can regain control over their mental health, understanding that there's no one-size-fits-all approach to depression treatment.

Antiarrhythmics

Antiarrhythmics are medications designed to address abnormal heart rhythms, also known as arrhythmias. These drugs play a crucial role in restoring the heart's normal rhythm and preventing potentially dangerous complications associated with irregular heartbeats. Understanding how antiarrhythmics function is essential for individuals with heart conditions or those at risk for arrhythmias.

The treatment of irregular heartbeats involves the use of antiarrhythmic medications. These drugs are complex and operate based on the Vaughan Williams (VW) classification system, introduced in 1970. The VW classification categorizes antiarrhythmics into five classes (I, II, III, IV, and V), each targeting different aspects of the heart's electrical system. These medications aim to inhibit ion channels in heart muscles, thereby minimizing excessive heartbeats.

Class I drugs, known as Sodium (Na+) Channel Blockers, include disopyramide, pilsicainide hydrochloride, and lidocaine. They function by inhibiting sodium ions from entering heart muscle, prolonging the action potential's duration, and extending the resting period for the next nerve impulse.

Class II drugs, Beta-blockers such as propranolol and atenolol, block both sodium and calcium ion channels while also regulating catecholamines, thereby controlling heart rate.

Class III drugs, including amiodarone, nifekalant, and dofetilide, extend the repolarization time by blocking potassium channels, thereby increasing the refractory period and delaying subsequent nerve impulses.

Class IV drugs, Slow Calcium (Ca2+) Channel Blockers like diltiazem and verapamil, reduce conduction via the AV node, shortening the cardiac action potential's next phase and inhibiting excessive excitement in heart muscle cells.

Class V drugs, categorized as Other Agents, have mechanisms not fitting into the previous classes. For instance, adenosine temporarily blocks the AV node by reducing cAMP levels, while digoxin increases vagal activity to reduce conductivity in the AV node.

In addition to medication, alternative medicine practitioners may explore natural remedies and lifestyle changes to manage arrhythmias, including dietary modifications, stress management techniques, and herbal supplements. Nurses and healthcare providers must grasp the mechanisms of action of antiarrhythmics to deliver quality care to patients with heart conditions, monitoring for signs of arrhythmias and ensuring appropriate treatment.

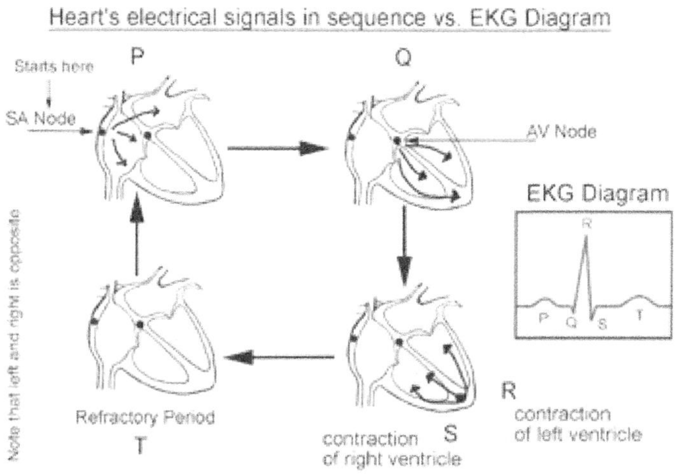

Visual animation illustration: http://www.nhlbi.nih.gov/health/dci/Diseases/hhw/hhw_electrical.html

In conclusion, antiarrhythmics are indispensable in managing abnormal heart rhythms and promoting heart health. Through education about these medications, individuals, healthcare providers, and alternative medicine practitioners can collaborate to optimize treatment plans and enhance overall well-being.

Analgesic

Analgesics, commonly known as painkillers, are medications used to alleviate pain and reduce inflammation by blocking pain signals transmitted to the brain. There are two primary types of analgesics: non-opioid analgesics, such as acetaminophen and nonsteroidal anti-inflammatory drugs (NSAIDs) like ibuprofen, and opioid analgesics, including codeine and morphine.

Non-opioid analgesics are typically employed for mild to moderate pain management, such as headaches, muscle aches, and arthritis. They are available over-the-counter and generally safe when used as directed. However, long-term use of NSAIDs can lead to adverse effects like stomach ulcers and kidney damage. Acetaminophen, a popular NSAID, acts on the COX enzyme responsible for prostaglandin synthesis, reducing pain, fever, and inflammation. However, its inhibition of COX-1 alongside COX-2 can lead to complications like liver damage.

Opioid analgesics target opioid receptors in the central nervous system and along intestinal nerves. Morphine and codeine, derived from the opium plant, act on mu-receptors to relieve pain. While highly effective, opioids carry a risk of addiction and overdose, making responsible use imperative. Physical dependence is also a concern with long-term opioid use. In low doses, codeine is used to suppress cough.

Alternative pain relief methods complement traditional analgesics and include acupuncture, massage therapy, herbal remedies, and mindfulness meditation. Numerous studies are currently demonstrating promising outcomes regarding the use of meditation in the treatment of chronic pain patients. Some individuals are successfully achieving mental relaxation and acquiring the ability to reduce reliance on painkillers. One contributing factor to the dependency caused by opiates is the suppression of endorphin production in the body when these medications are introduced into the system.

In conclusion, analgesics are essential tools for pain management, improving individuals' quality of life. By understanding their mechanisms and using them responsibly, individuals can find relief from pain while minimizing risks and complications. Working closely with healthcare providers identifies the most suitable pain management approach.

Medication for Cancer

Cancer remains a formidable adversary, affecting countless individuals worldwide. Medications play an important role in combating this disease among the arsenal of treatments available. This section delves into the diverse types of medications employed in cancer treatment, elucidating their mechanisms of action and potential side effects.

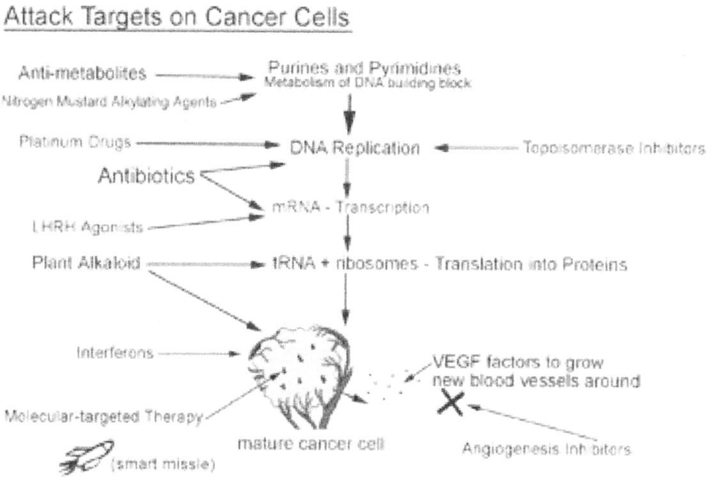

Killing Cancer Cells Drugs

1. **Nitrogen Mustard Alkylating Agents*:** These agents attach

alkyl groups to DNA, specifically the guanine base, impeding DNA replication. Examples include melphalan, cyclophosphamide, and nimustine hydrochloride. Replication becomes impeded as DNA strands are essentially immobilized, unable to uncoil properly. Examples of such agents include melphalan, cyclophosphamide, and nimustine hydrochloride.

*These agents gained notoriety as chemical weapons during World War I under the name "mustard gas.

2. **Anti-metabolites:** Drugs like methotrexate hinder DNA and RNA synthesis by impeding the incorporation of building blocks into nucleic acids. Methotrexate, fluorouracil, and mercaptopurine are notable examples. Methotrexate bears a structural resemblance to folic acid and acts as an antagonist by binding to the enzyme. Similarly, fluorouracil impedes thymidylate synthase, while mercaptopurine competes with normal purine to form AMP and GMP. To elaborate, fluorouracil inhibits the function of thymidylate synthase, an enzyme crucial for synthesizing thymidine monophosphate (dTMP), a component of DNA. Meanwhile, mercaptopurine competes with natural purines to form AMP and GMP, essential components of DNA and RNA. In DNA, there are two types of nucleotide bases: purines (adenine and guanine) and pyrimidines (cytosine and thymine). These bases pair up to form the building blocks of DNA strands.

3. **Antibiotics as Chemotherapeutic Agents:** Mitomycin C forms crosslinks with DNA, while doxorubicin disrupts DNA replication. Both are used in cancer treatment.

4. **Plant Alkaloids:** Vincristine, derived from the vinca plant,

disrupts microtubule formation, preventing cell division. Paclitaxel stabilizes microtubules, inhibiting their degradation.

5. **Platinum-containing Drugs:** Cisplatin binds DNA, inducing apoptosis. Carboplatin and nedaplatin are other examples.

6. **Hydrolysis Enzymes:** L-asparaginase targets acute lymphoblastic leukemia by depleting circulating asparagine, causing leukemic cell death due to nutrient starvation.

7. **Endocrine Therapy with Luteinizing Hormone-Releasing Hormone (LHRH) Agonists:** Hormone-responsive cancers, such as breast cancer, can be treated with tamoxifen, exemestane, or leuprorelin acetate, which inhibit estrogen production or action. Tamoxifen functions as an antagonist by binding to estrogen receptors, thereby preventing estrogen from binding to receptors in breast tissue. On the other hand, Exemestane operates by permanently binding to the enzyme responsible for converting androgens into estrogens. Another example is leuprorelin acetate, which acts on pituitary GnRH receptors, leading to the downregulation of luteinizing hormone (LH) and follicle-stimulating hormone (FSH) secretion. In women, this treatment is used to address breast and ovarian cancer**, while in men, it suppresses testosterone production to manage advanced prostate cancer.

**Cancer cells, despite sharing common names such as breast cancer, can exhibit diverse behaviors. Therefore, breast cancer is further categorized into hormone-responsive and hormone-nonresponsive types.

8. **Topoisomerase Inhibitors:** Drugs like irinotecan and etopo-

side impede DNA unwinding and replication by inhibiting topoisomerase enzymes. Topoisomerases play a vital role in DNA replication and transcription by cutting and reannealing*** DNA strands and unwinding them. These enzymes are indispensable for cell growth and protein synthesis. Drugs that inhibit topoisomerases prevent DNA from unwinding, thereby blocking DNA replication. Irinotecan acts as a topoisomerase 1 inhibitor, inhibiting the cutting of one strand of a DNA double helix. Conversely, etoposide serves as a topoisomerase 2 inhibitor, inhibiting the cutting of both strands of a DNA double helix.

***Reanneal refers to the process of forming duplex DNA or combining two single strands of DNA into double-stranded DNA.

9. **Angiogenesis Inhibitors:** Bevacizumab and carboxyamidotriazole prevent angiogenesis by inhibiting Vascular Endothelial Growth Factor (VEGF) from binding to endothelial cell receptors. Solid masses of cancer require nutrients to support their growth, prompting cancer cells to induce the formation of new blood vessels through a process called angiogenesis. By growing these new blood vessels, cancer cells ensure a continuous supply of nutrients. Antiangiogenic drugs function by preventing the binding of Vascular Endothelial Growth Factor (VEGF) to receptors on endothelial cells. Since endothelial cells are responsible for forming new blood vessel walls, inhibiting this process hinders the growth of blood vessels around cancerous masses. This treatment capitalizes on the fact that the adult body typically forms new vessels only during active tissue repair. Examples of antiangiogenic drugs include bevacizumab and carboxyamidotriazole.

10. **Interferons (IFN):** Naturally occurring proteins, Interferons, including IFN-alpha, IFN-beta, and IFN-gamma, are naturally occurring proteins that stimulate the immune system to recognize and eradicate cancerous cells. Drugs like Multiferon and Imidazoquinoline harness the immune-boosting capabilities of interferons in cancer treatment. Produced by various cells in the body, interferons act as a signaling system, aiding the immune system in targeting and neutralizing threats. Multiferon, for instance, is employed in treating cutaneous melanoma, capitalizing on interferons' immune-enhancing properties.

Similarly, compounds such as Imidazoquinoline can trigger the production of IFN-alpha, further bolstering the immune response against cancer. While these medications offer significant promise, they are not without side effects. Patients undergoing cancer treatment should collaborate closely with healthcare providers to tailor an effective treatment plan, optimizing outcomes while managing potential adverse effects.

Molecular-targeted Therapy for Cancer

Molecular-targeted therapy represents a specialized approach to combatting cancer by zeroing in on specific molecules within cancer cells. Unlike conventional chemotherapy, which can affect healthy cells along with cancerous ones, targeted therapy aims to disrupt the signaling pathways that drive cancer growth while minimizing damage to normal tissues.

1. **Gefitinib:**

This medication functions as an inhibitor of epidermal growth factor receptors (EGFR), which are crucial for cell proliferation and DNA synthesis. By targeting EGFR, gefitinib disrupts the signaling pathways that promote the growth of malignant cells.

2. **Trastuzumab:**

Trastuzumab is a monoclonal antibody designed to target the HER2/neu receptor, which is often overexpressed in certain types of cancer cells, particularly breast cancer. By binding to HER2/neu receptors on the cell membrane, trastuzumab interferes with intercellular communication, impeding cancer cell growth and survival.

3. **Imatinib Mesilate (Gleevec):**

Imatinib is a tyrosine kinase inhibitor used primarily in the treatment of chronic myelogenous leukemia (CML). It works by inhibiting the activity of the BCR-ABL protein, which arises from a chromosomal mutation characteristic of CML. BCR-ABL is an abnormal tyrosine kinase that activates various cell cycle-controlling proteins and enzymes, leading to uncontrolled cell division. By blocking the action of BCR-ABL, imatinib helps to restore normal cell growth regulation and control the progression of leukemia.

5

Chapter 5: Herbal Remedies and Alternative Medicine

Overview of Herbal Medicine

Herbal medicine, also referred to as botanical medicine or phytotherapy, encompasses a traditional healing approach that relies on plants and their extracts to address a wide range of health conditions. This age-old practice has been deeply rooted in cultures worldwide for centuries and continues to be embraced by various segments of society, including health-conscious individuals, nurses, patients, alternative medicine practitioners, and other healthcare professionals.

Central to the concept of herbal medicine is the belief in the therapeutic properties of natural compounds found within plants. These bioactive compounds, such as alkaloids, flavonoids, and terpenes, are thought to exert healing effects on the body, promoting recovery, alleviating symptoms, and enhancing overall health and vitality. Notably, many pharmaceutical drugs have their origins in botanical sources, exemplified by aspirin derived from willow bark and paclitaxel, a chemotherapy drug sourced from the Pacific yew tree.

An inherent advantage of herbal medicine lies in its perceived natural and holistic approach to healthcare. Many individuals gravitate towards herbal remedies due to the perception of their safety and reduced risk of adverse effects compared to synthetic pharmaceuticals. Moreover, herbal medicine often offers a more accessible and cost-effective alternative to prescription medications.

However, it is essential to recognize that herbal medicine carries its own set of risks and considerations. Despite their natural origins, certain herbs may interact with medications or pose hazards when consumed in excessive quantities. Therefore, consulting with a qualified healthcare provider before initiating any herbal treatment is crucial to ensure safety and efficacy.

In addition to conventional herbal practices, Traditional Chinese Medicine (TCM) represents a rich and longstanding tradition of herbal healing. TCM employs a vast array of herbs and plant extracts, often formulated into complex herbal combinations known as herbal formulas. These formulations are meticulously crafted to rebalance the body's vital energy, or qi, and address specific health imbalances based on TCM diagnostic principles.

Let's explore the historical roots of herbal medicine, learn the diverse applications of medicinal plants in healing, discuss common herbal remedies for various health conditions, and examine both the potential benefits and risks associated with herbal medicine. By gaining insight into the fundamentals of herbal medicine, individuals can make informed decisions regarding their health and well-being, incorporating traditional wisdom alongside modern healthcare practices.

Common Herbal Remedies and Their Uses

Herbal remedies have been used for centuries to treat various ailments and promote overall well-being. In this section, we will explore some of the most common herbal remedies and their uses.

1. **Echinacea:** Echinacea is a popular herb known for its immune-boosting properties. It is often used to prevent and treat colds and flu. Echinacea can help reduce the severity and duration of symptoms associated with these illnesses.
2. **Ginger:** Ginger is well-known for its anti-inflammatory and digestive properties. It can help alleviate nausea, indigestion, and bloating. Ginger can also be used to reduce muscle pain and soreness.
3. **Peppermint:** Peppermint is commonly used to relieve digestive issues such as gas, bloating, and indigestion. It can also help alleviate headaches and improve mental clarity. Peppermint oil can be applied topically to soothe sore muscles and joints.
4. **Valerian:** Valerian is a natural sedative that can help promote relaxation and improve sleep quality. It is often used to treat insomnia and anxiety. Valerian can also help reduce menstrual cramps and muscle tension.
5. **Turmeric:** Turmeric is a potent anti-inflammatory herb that can help reduce pain and inflammation in the body. It is often used to treat conditions such as arthritis, joint pain, and digestive issues. Turmeric can also help improve cognitive function and boost the immune system.

These are just a few examples of common herbal remedies and their uses. It is important to consult with a healthcare provider before using any herbal remedy, especially if you are pregnant, nursing, or taking medication. Incorporating herbal remedies into your healthcare routine can be a natural and effective way to promote health and well-being.

Common Herbal Remedies using Traditional Chinese Medicine (TCM) and Their Uses

Traditional Chinese Medicine (TCM) boasts a rich legacy of herbal healing, rooted in centuries of empirical knowledge and holistic principles. In TCM, herbs are meticulously selected and combined into complex formulations known as herbal formulas, with each herb chosen for its specific therapeutic properties and synergistic effects. These herbal remedies are often utilized to restore balance to the body's vital energy, or qi, and address a wide array of health concerns. Below are some common herbal remedies used in TCM along with their traditional uses:

1. Ginseng (Ren Shen)

Traditional Use: Ginseng is prized for its adaptogenic properties, helping to enhance vitality, boost energy levels, and strengthen the body's resilience to stress. It is often prescribed for fatigue, weakness, and overall debility.

2. Astragalus (Huang Qi)

Traditional Use: Astragalus is renowned for its immune-boosting effects, promoting resistance to infections and supporting immune function. It is commonly used to prevent and treat respiratory infections, such as colds and flu.

3. Ginger (Sheng Jiang)

Traditional Use: Ginger is valued for its warming and digestive properties, aiding in the relief of nausea, indigestion, and abdominal discomfort. It is also used to promote circulation and alleviate cold symptoms.

4. Licorice Root (Gan Cao)

Traditional Use: Licorice root is known for its harmonizing and soothing effects on the body. It is frequently included in herbal formulas to enhance the flavor and balance the actions of other herbs. Additionally, licorice root is used to alleviate coughs, soothe sore throats, and support adrenal function.

5. Chinese Angelica Root (Dang Gui)

Traditional Use: Chinese angelica root is esteemed for its blood-nourishing and circulation-promoting properties. It is commonly prescribed for conditions related to blood deficiency, such as irregular menstruation, anemia, and postpartum recovery.

6. Coptis Root (Huang Lian)

Traditional Use: Coptis root possesses strong antimicrobial and anti-inflammatory properties, making it a valuable remedy for gastrointestinal infections, diarrhea, and inflammatory conditions of the digestive tract.

7. Rehmannia Root (Shu Di Huang)

Traditional Use: Rehmannia root is revered for its kidney-tonifying and blood-enriching actions. It is frequently utilized in formulas for nourishing the yin, replenishing vital essence, and addressing conditions such as chronic fatigue, insomnia, and menopausal symptoms.

8. Schisandra Berry (Wu Wei Zi)

Traditional Use: Schisandra berry is known for its adaptogenic and liver-protective properties. It is used to enhance endurance, combat fatigue, and support liver function, making it beneficial for individuals experiencing stress or liver-related disorders.

These are just a few examples of the countless herbal remedies employed in Traditional Chinese Medicine. TCM practitioners carefully tailor herbal formulas to suit each individual's unique constitution and health needs, emphasizing the importance of personalized treatment approaches. While TCM herbal remedies have been utilized for centuries, it is advisable to consult with a qualified TCM practitioner or healthcare provider before incorporating these remedies into your healthcare regimen.

Combining Conventional and Alternative Medicine

The integration of conventional medicine and alternative therapies has become increasingly popular in recent years. This approach, known as integrative medicine, combines the best of both worlds to provide comprehensive care for patients.

Conventional medicine, often referred to as Western medicine, is based on scientific evidence and uses pharmaceutical drugs and surgical procedures to treat illnesses and diseases. While conventional medicine is highly effective in many cases, it often focuses on treating symptoms rather than addressing the root cause of the problem. Alternative medicine, on the other hand, takes a more holistic approach to healing, considering the mind, body, and spirit as interconnected parts of a whole.

By combining conventional and alternative medicine, patients can benefit from the strengths of both approaches. Conventional medicine can provide quick relief for acute conditions, while alternative therapies such as acupuncture, herbal medicine, and yoga can promote long-term healing and prevention. Integrative medicine also allows for a more personalized approach to treatment, taking into account each individual's unique needs and preferences.

For health-conscious individuals, nurses, patients, and alternative medicine practitioners, understanding the principles of integrative medicine can help improve outcomes and promote overall well-being. By working together with a healthcare team that includes both conventional and alternative practitioners, patients can receive the best of both worlds and achieve optimal health.

6

Chapter 6: Pharmacology and Mental Health

Navigating Mental Health During Illness: Supporting Ourselves and Our Loved Ones

When facing illness or health challenges, it's important to recognize the impact they can have on mental health and behavior. Illness often brings about a range of emotions, from fear and anxiety to frustration and sadness. These feelings can lead to changes in behavior, such as withdrawal, irritability, or difficulty concentrating. To improve mental health during these times, it's crucial to prioritize self-care. This includes maintaining healthy habits like regular exercise, adequate sleep, and balanced nutrition, as well as seeking support from loved ones or mental health professionals when needed. When caring for someone who is sick, extra patience and understanding are essential. Providing emotional support, actively listening, and offering reassurance can make a significant difference in their well-being. Additionally, taking breaks and seeking support for

yourself as a caregiver is important for maintaining your own mental health and resilience. **For long-term care of someone, it's important to ask for help from other people, as care giving can be exhausting.** Seeking assistance not only ensures better care for your loved one but also helps you take care of yourself. Through compassion, understanding, and self-care, we can navigate the challenges of illness while supporting ourselves and our loved ones effectively.

Psychotropic Medications

Psychotropic medications are drugs that affect the mind, emotions, and behavior. These medications are commonly used to treat mental health conditions such as depression, anxiety, bipolar disorder, and schizophrenia. They work by altering the levels of neurotransmitters in the brain, which are chemicals that help nerve cells communicate with each other.

Health-conscious individuals should be aware of the potential benefits and risks of psychotropic medications. While these medications can be effective in treating mental health conditions, they can also have side effects and interactions with other drugs. It is important to work closely with a healthcare provider to find the right medication and dosage for your individual needs.

Nurses and healthcare workers play a crucial role in administering psychotropic medications to patients. They must have a thorough understanding of the different types of psychotropic medications, how they work, and how to safely administer them. Nurses also play a key role in monitoring patients for any potential side effects or adverse reactions to the medications.

Patients who are prescribed psychotropic medications should

be proactive in their treatment. It is important to follow the prescribed dosage and schedule, as well as to communicate any concerns or side effects to your healthcare provider. Patients should also be aware of the potential risks of abruptly stopping psychotropic medications, as this can lead to withdrawal symptoms.

Alternative medicine practitioners may also work with patients who are taking psychotropic medications. It is important for these practitioners to have a basic understanding of how these medications work and how they may interact with other treatments. Collaboration between conventional and alternative healthcare providers can help ensure the best possible outcomes for patients.

In conclusion, psychotropic medications play a vital role in the treatment of mental health conditions. By understanding how these medications work and working closely with healthcare providers, individuals can safely and effectively manage their mental health.

Impact of Drugs on Mental Health

In contemporary society, drug use has become increasingly prevalent, whether for medicinal purposes or recreational enjoyment. Yet, the profound impact of drugs on mental health is often overlooked. In this discussion, we will delve into how various drugs affect the mind and the potential repercussions for mental well-being.

Alcohol stands as one of the most common substances with a significant impact on mental health. While occasional consumption is common, excessive intake can precipitate depression, anxiety, and other mood disorders. Moreover, alcohol impairs judgment and decision-making, fostering risky behaviors that further compound mental health challenges.

Stimulants, including amphetamines and cocaine, represent another class of drugs known to influence mental health. Though they may temporarily elevate energy and alertness, they can also induce paranoia, hallucinations, and mood instability. Prolonged use often leads to addiction and exacerbates mental health issues.

Conversely, certain medications used to manage mental health conditions, such as antidepressants and antipsychotics, can positively impact mental well-being when administered as prescribed. However, misuse or sudden cessation of these medications can trigger withdrawal symptoms and worsen mental health symptoms.

It is imperative for individuals invested in health, including nurses, caregivers, patients, practitioners of alternative medicine, and healthcare professionals, to recognize the profound impact of drugs on mental health. By comprehending the diverse effects of different drugs on the psyche, we can make informed choices regarding their utilization and advocate for safer drug practices. Remember, prioritizing mental health is as crucial as attending to physical health for overall well-being.

Regarding the mechanism of drugs penetrating the blood-brain barrier and affecting the brain, it's worth mentioning that substances can cross this barrier through various mechanisms. Lipophilic drugs, for instance, can passively diffuse through the lipid-rich cell membranes of brain capillary endothelial cells. Additionally, certain drugs utilize specific transport mechanisms, such as carrier-mediated transport or receptor-mediated transcytosis, to cross the blood-brain barrier. Understanding these mechanisms can shed light on how drugs exert their effects on the brain and influence mental health.

Integrative Approaches to Mental Health

In our modern, hectic world, mental health challenges are increasingly prevalent. From common issues like anxiety and depression to more complex conditions such as bipolar disorder and schizophrenia, many individuals find themselves grappling with the pressures of daily life. While conventional pharmaceutical treatments play a vital role in managing mental health disorders, there is a growing interest in integrative approaches that adopt a holistic perspective on mental well-being.

Integrative approaches to mental health prioritize treating the entire individual, rather than solely addressing isolated symptoms of a particular disorder. This approach may involve a blend of traditional pharmaceutical interventions, alternative therapies, lifestyle adjustments, and holistic practices like meditation and yoga. By digging into the root causes of mental health issues and nurturing overall wellness, integrative strategies offer a more comprehensive and impactful treatment framework for individuals navigating mental health challenges.

A broad spectrum of individuals, including health-conscious individuals, nurses, caregivers, patients, practitioners of alternative medicine, and healthcare professionals, can benefit from exploring integrative approaches to mental health. By acquainting themselves with the diverse array of treatment modalities available, individuals can collaborate with their healthcare providers to craft personalized treatment plans tailored to their unique needs and preferences. Whether embracing mindfulness practices as part of daily routines, exploring the potential benefits of herbal supplements, or venturing into realms like acupuncture or massage therapy, there exists a plethora of avenues to bolster mental well-being beyond traditional pharmaceutical avenues.

By exploring the multifaceted realm of treatment options and embracing the potential advantages of a holistic approach to mental health, individuals empower themselves to make informed decisions about their mental healthcare journey.

7

Chapter 7: Pharmacology in Everyday Life

Medication Safety Tips

Ensuring the safe use of medication is paramount for safeguarding overall health and well-being. Whether you're a conscientious health enthusiast, a diligent nurse, a vigilant patient, an alternative medicine practitioner, or any other healthcare professional, adhering to these medication safety guidelines can mitigate the risks of harmful drug interactions and adverse effects.

1. **Seek Professional Guidance:** Always consult with a qualified healthcare professional before initiating any new medication or supplement regimen. They can provide vital insights regarding potential side effects, drug interactions, and appropriate dosages tailored to your needs.
2. **Maintain a Comprehensive Medication Record:** Keep a meticulously curated inventory of all medications you're

currently taking, encompassing prescription drugs, over-the-counter medications, supplements, and herbal remedies. Regularly update this list and furnish it to your healthcare provider for informed decision-making.

3. **Adhere to Prescribed Dosages:** Strictly adhere to the dosing instructions provided by your healthcare provider. Deviating from the recommended dosage, whether by excess or deficit, can precipitate severe health repercussions. Additionally, consult with your doctor before making any changes to your dosage, and be vigilant in reporting any severe side effects.
4. **Exercise Caution with Drug Interactions:** Stay vigilant about potential interactions between medications. Certain drug combinations can engender adverse effects or compromise the efficacy of one or both drugs. Always confer with your healthcare provider prior to co-administering medications.
5. **Store Medications Appropriately:** Store medications in their original containers, shielded from excessive heat, moisture, and direct sunlight. Refrain from using medications that have exceeded their expiration date or exhibit alterations in color, texture, or odor.
6. **Exercise Prudence with Online Pharmacies:** Exercise discernment when procuring medications from online pharmacies. Prioritize reputable sources and validate the authenticity of the pharmacy before consummating any transactions.
7. **Stay Attuned to Allergic Reactions:** Remain vigilant for potential allergic reactions to medications. If you encounter any anomalous symptoms subsequent to medication intake, such as rash, swelling, or respiratory distress,

promptly seek medical intervention.

8. **Monitoring IV Medications in Hospital Care:** During hospitalization, vigilantly monitor and document intravenous (IV) medications. Since IV regimens can change daily, accurately recording the name and dosage of each injection is essential. This proactive measure helps prevent medication errors and ensures consistent care, aiding in understanding the progress and condition of your loved ones throughout their hospital stay.

By adhering steadfastly to these medication safety guidelines, you fortify the efficacy and security of your treatment regimen. Remember, your health constitutes your most invaluable asset, necessitating judiciousness in all facets of medication usage.

Responsible Medication Use

Responsible Medication Management is paramount for safeguarding your health and overall well-being. This section will discuss the significance of adhering to prescribed medication regimens, comprehending potential side effects, and taking proactive measures to manage your medications effectively.

For individuals who prioritize their health, understanding their prescribed medications and their potential impacts on both body and mind is imperative. By acquiring knowledge about the potential benefits and risks associated with various medications, informed decisions can be made regarding one's healthcare.

Nurses and healthcare professionals hold a pivotal role in patient education concerning medications. By furnishing patients with clear instructions and addressing any inquiries they may harbor, nurses contribute significantly to fostering responsible medication use and enhancing patient outcomes.

Patients are encouraged to actively engage in their healthcare journey by meticulously adhering to the directives provided by their healthcare providers and voicing any queries or concerns that may arise. Effective communication regarding side effects or apprehensions with healthcare providers ensures the safety and efficacy of the treatment plan.

Alternative medicine practitioners should exercise vigilance regarding potential interactions between conventional medications and herbal supplements. An understanding of how different treatments may interact empowers practitioners to guide their patients towards avoiding adverse effects and attaining improved health outcomes.

In essence, responsible medication management stands as a cornerstone of maintaining optimal health and well-being. Through informed decision-making, proactive engagement, and collaborative efforts with healthcare providers, individuals can ensure the safe and effective utilization of medications. Always remember that your health lies within your hands; thus, exercising prudence and responsibility in your medication regimen is paramount.

Advocating for Your Health

In our fast-paced world, it is easy to overlook the importance of advocating for our health. As health-conscious individuals, nurses, health takers, patients, alternative medicine practitioners, and health workers, it is crucial that we take an active role in managing our well-being. This includes being informed about our medications and understanding how they affect our bodies and minds.

One key way to advocate for your health is to educate yourself about pharmacology for everyday people. Understanding how drugs work in the body can help you make informed decisions about your healthcare. By learning about the potential side effects, interactions, and contraindications of medications, you can work with your healthcare provider to develop a treatment plan tailored to your needs.

Another important aspect of advocating for your health is communication. It is essential to have open and honest conversations with your healthcare provider about your concerns, preferences, and goals for treatment. By actively participating in these discussions, you can ensure that your voice is heard and that your healthcare decisions align with your values and beliefs.

Additionally, it is important to take an active role in monitoring your health and seeking out alternative medicine options when appropriate. By exploring complementary therapies and lifestyle changes, you can optimize your health and well-being holistically.

In conclusion, advocating for your health is vital to self-care and well-being. By educating yourself about pharmacology, communicating effectively with your healthcare provider, and exploring alternative medicine options, you can take control of your health and empower yourself to make informed decisions about your care. Remember, your health is your most valuable asset – so make it a priority!

8

Chapter 8: Conclusion and Future of Pharmacology

Recap of Key Concepts

As we wrap up this section on how drugs affect your body and mind, let's take a moment to recap some of the key concepts we've discussed so far. Whether you are a health-conscious individual, nurse, patient, alternative medicine practitioner, or any other health worker, understanding the basics of pharmacology is crucial for making informed decisions about your health and well-being.

First and foremost, it's important to remember that drugs can have a profound impact on both your body and mind. From over-the-counter medications to prescription drugs, each substance you put into your body has the potential to produce a range of effects, both positive and negative. It's essential to be aware of how different drugs work and the potential risks and benefits associated with their use.

We've also discussed the importance of proper medication

management, including understanding dosage instructions, potential interactions with other drugs or substances, and how to recognize and report any adverse reactions. Being proactive about your health and asking questions about your medications can help prevent potentially harmful outcomes.

Additionally, we've touched on the role of alternative medicine in pharmacology and how natural remedies and supplements can also impact your body and mind. It's crucial to approach these options with caution and consult with a healthcare professional before incorporating them into your treatment plan.

In conclusion, the world of pharmacology is vast and complex, but by understanding the key concepts we've covered, you can navigate it more confidently and make informed decisions about your health. Remember to always prioritize your well-being and seek out reliable sources of information when it comes to medication and treatment options. Your health is worth it.

Emerging Trends in Pharmacology

In the dynamic realm of pharmacology, new trends continually shape the landscape of drug development, prescription, and consumption. It is essential for health-conscious individuals, including nurses, patients, alternative medicine practitioners, and healthcare workers, to remain abreast of these trends to make informed decisions about health and well-being.

Personalized Medicine: Among the most impactful trends is the ascent of personalized medicine. This paradigm considers an individual's genetic makeup, lifestyle, and environmental factors to tailor drug treatments uniquely to their requirements. By scrutinizing a person's genetic profile, healthcare providers can ascertain the most suitable and safe medications, mitigating the risk of adverse reactions and enhancing overall outcomes.

Integration of Natural and Alternative Remedies: Another notable trend is the increasing utilization of natural and alternative remedies. With a mounting interest in holistic health and wellness, many individuals are exploring herbal supplements, acupuncture, and other alternative therapies for various conditions. While scientific evidence may vary, these methods can be effective for some and often entail fewer side effects.

Innovative Drug Delivery Systems: Moreover, the evolution of novel drug delivery systems is transforming medication administration. From transdermal patches to implantable devices, these advanced technologies enhance patient compliance and outcomes by ensuring precise dosing and targeted drug delivery to specific body regions.

AI-Assisted Drug Discovery: Additionally, the integration of artificial intelligence (AI) in drug discovery has revolutionized the pharmaceutical landscape. AI algorithms analyze vast datasets to identify potential drug candidates, predict their efficacy and safety profiles, and even custom-design molecules tailored to specific therapeutic targets. This approach accelerates drug development, streamlines clinical trials, and enhances the efficiency of bringing new medications to market.

By staying informed about these evolving trends in pharmacology, individuals can navigate healthcare decisions with greater confidence and knowledge. Whether seeking treatment for a specific ailment or striving to maintain overall well-being, understanding these trends empowers individuals to engage with pharmaceutical advancements effectively and optimize their health outcomes.

Personalized Medicine and Its Impact on Healthcare

Personalized medicine, also known as precision medicine, is at the forefront of healthcare innovation. It offers tailored treatment strategies based on an individual's genetic makeup, lifestyle, and environment. This approach enables healthcare providers to prescribe medications and therapies customized to each patient, maximizing efficacy while minimizing adverse effects.

The advent of custom-designed drugs is a significant part of this transformation. These drugs are designed to mimic the pharmacological effects of original drugs, thereby providing more effective and personalized treatment options. The use of AI in personalized medicine is also on the rise. AI can analyze large datasets to identify patterns and relationships, which can help in predicting individual health risks and outcomes. This allows for more personalized treatment plans, better clinical decisions, and ultimately improved patient care. The future of healthcare personalization will require connected tools and data, widespread automation, an abundance of data, and proactive treatment.

For health-conscious individuals, personalized medicine holds the promise of more targeted and effective treatments, fostering improved health outcomes. Armed with insights into how drugs interact with their bodies on a molecular level, individuals can make informed decisions about their healthcare and take proactive steps to manage their well-being.

Nurses and healthcare professionals play a pivotal role in implementing personalized medicine, facilitating the collection and analysis of patient data, interpreting genetic test results, and devising personalized treatment plans. Their expertise ensures patients receive optimal and tailored care, optimizing treatment efficacy and patient satisfaction.

Patients benefit from personalized medicine by receiving treatments precisely tailored to their needs, enhancing treatment success rates and reducing the risk of adverse reactions. By collaborating closely with healthcare providers to develop personalized treatment plans, patients assume greater control over their health and enhance their quality of life.

Alternative medicine practitioners can also embrace personalized medicine, offering patients a holistic and individualized approach to healthcare. By integrating traditional healing modalities with state-of-the-art genetic and pharmacological therapies, alternative medicine practitioners provide patients with comprehensive and personalized treatment plans addressing their unique needs.

Personalized medicine represents a paradigm shift in healthcare, offering a more targeted, effective, and individualized approach to treatment. By leveraging the synergies of pharmacology and genetics, healthcare providers can enhance patient outcomes, reduce healthcare costs, and ultimately save lives.

Conclusion

Our minds wield the greatest healing power of all. Have you ever pondered the placebo effect? It's a fascinating phenomenon where patients experience tangible improvements despite receiving inert "sugar pills" with no therapeutic properties, all because they are unaware of their true nature. And did you know that fear can precipitate health issues, and in extreme cases, even lead to death? Consider the chilling tale from World War II: a blindfolded prisoner, convinced he would bleed to death from a mere scratch, succumbed to his own terror upon hearing the drip of a faucet. These anecdotes underscore the profound influence our minds hold over our well-being.

Your thoughts can chart diverse courses of action. Upon completing this book, I trust you will gain fresh insights into the intricate biochemistry unfolding within your body, fostering a deeper appreciation for life itself. These biochemical reactions transcend mere chemistry; they signify a harmonious collaboration between you and your body in the fight against illness. Indeed, you are the ultimate line of defense.

Prioritize your physical well-being. Incorporating a new exercise routine can boost energy levels significantly. You don't need strenuous workouts or gym memberships; consistency in exercise and balanced nutrition is key. Consider adding meditation to your routine; it's a workout for the mind! Experience the powerful benefits of nurturing both body and mind for enhanced health and vitality.

Appendix I: Prescription abbreviations used by medical professionals

As health-conscious individuals, patients, nurses, and alternative medicine practitioners, it is essential to have a basic understanding of prescription abbreviations commonly used by medical professionals. This knowledge can help you better understand your medications, communicate effectively with healthcare providers, and ensure safe and effective treatment.

Here are some of the most common prescription abbreviations you may encounter:

1. PO - By mouth (per os): This abbreviation indicates that a medication should be taken orally, or by mouth. It is one of the most common routes of drug administration.
2. QD - Once a day (quaque die): This abbreviation indicates that a medication should be taken once daily.
3. BID - Twice a day (bis in die): This abbreviation indicates that a medication should be taken twice daily.
4. TID - Three times a day (ter in die): This abbreviation indicates that a medication should be taken three times daily.
5. PRN - As needed (pro re nata): This abbreviation indicates that a medication should be taken only when needed,

rather than on a regular schedule.

6. QID - Four times a day (quater in die): This abbreviation indicates that a medication should be taken four times daily.
7. IM - Intramuscular: This abbreviation indicates that a medication should be administered into a muscle, rather than orally or intravenously.

Understanding these abbreviations can help you follow your healthcare provider's instructions more accurately and ensure the safe and effective use of medications. You can familiarize yourself with the frequently used Latin-based abbreviations on your prescription, which your doctor provided following a medical appointment.

Abbreviation / Meaning / Latin

Aa /of each/ ana
Ad/ up to / ad
a.c. /Before meals/ Ante cibum
a.d./ right ear/ aurio dextra
ad.lib. /use as much as one wants /Ad libitum
admov/ apply / admove
agit/ stir or shake / agita
alt. h. / every other hour / alternis horis
a.m. / morning, before noon / alternis meridiem
aq. /Water /Aqua
b.i.d. /Twice a day /Bis in die
b.i.n. /Twice a night/ Bis in noctus
c / with bar on top /With /Cum
c / food / cibos
cap. /Capsule /Capula

cc / with food / cum cibos
cr., crm/ cream
cf / with food /
d /Day /Dies
daw /Dispense as written(no generic)
div. /Divide /Divide
eq.pts. /Equal parts /Equalis parties
gtt or gt /Drop /Gutta
h. /Hour /Hora
h.s. (hs) /Bedtime /Hora somni
ID / intradermal
I.M. /Into the muscle
I.V. /Into the vein
IVP / intravenous push
mg /Milligram
ml /Milliliter
no. /Number /Numero
noxt /At night
o. /Pint /Octarius
O.D. /Right eye /Oculo dextro
O.S. /Left eye /Oculo sinistro
O.U. /In each eye /Oculo utro
p.c. /After meals /Post cibum
p.m./ evening or afternoon / post meridiem
p.o. /By mouth /Per os
p.r.n. /As needed /Pre re nata
pulv / powder / pulvis
pil /Pill /Pilula
q 1 d /Every day /Quaque 1 die
q 1 w /Once a week
q 3 h /Every 3 hours /Quaque 3 hora

q.i.d. /4 times a day /Quarter in die
q.o.d. /Every other day
q.s. /Sufficient quantity /Quantum sufficiat
qAM/ Every morning
qd /Daily /Quaque die
qh /Every hour /Quaque hora
R / rectal
Rep / repeat / repetatur
s /Without Sine
s.i.d. /Once a day /Semel in die
s.l. /Under the tongue
Sig., S. /Write on the label /Signa
stat /Immediately /Statim
tab /Tablet /Tabella
tbsp /Tablespoon
tid /3 times a day /Ter in die
top / topical
tr, tinc / tincture
tsp /Teaspoon
ut dict /As directed by doctor
ung / ointment / unguentum
U.S.P / United States Pharmacopoeia
vag / vaginally
w / with
w/o / without
X / times
Y.O. /years old

Appendix II: Glossary of Pharmacology Terms

In the world of pharmacology, understanding the terminology is essential for comprehending how drugs affect the body and mind. This glossary provides definitions for key terms that you may encounter when discussing medication and its effects.

1. **Absorption:** The process by which a drug enters the bloodstream and reaches its target site in the body.
2. **Bioavailability**: The proportion of a drug that enters the circulation when introduced into the body and is able to have an active effect.
3. **Dosage**: The amount of a drug that is prescribed to be taken at one time or over a specific period.
4. **Metabolism**: The process by which the body breaks down drugs into smaller molecules that can be eliminated from the body.
5. **Side effects**: Unintended effects of a drug that may occur in addition to its desired therapeutic effects.
6. **Tolerance**: The body's decreased response to a drug over time, requiring higher doses to achieve the same effect.
7. **Withdrawal**: The physical and psychological symptoms that occur when a drug is discontinued after prolonged use.
8. **Over-the-counter (OTC)**: Medications that can be pur-

chased without a prescription and are generally considered safe for self-administration.

9. **Placebo**: A substance that has no therapeutic effect but may produce a psychological benefit when administered as if it were a real drug.
10. **Pharmacokinetics**: The study of how drugs are absorbed, distributed, metabolized, and excreted by the body.
11. **Efficacy**: This refers to the ability of a drug to produce a desired effect.
12. **Potency** refers to the strength or effectiveness of a drug, typically measured in milligrams, needed to produce a specific therapeutic effect.
13. **Adverse Effect**: Undesirable and unintended effects of a drug that occur at normal doses during treatment.
14. **Half-Life**: The time it takes for the concentration of a drug in the bloodstream to reduce by half.
15. **Route of Administration**: The method by which a drug is introduced into the body, such as oral, intravenous, topical, or inhalation.
16. **Receptor**: A protein molecule in a cell or on its surface with which a drug interacts to produce its pharmacological effects.
17. **Therapeutic Index**: The ratio between the dose of a drug that produces the desired therapeutic effect and the dose that produces toxic effects.

By familiarizing yourself with these terms, you can better understand how drugs work and make informed decisions about your health and medication. Whether you are a health-conscious individual, nurse, patient, alternative medicine practitioner, or health worker, this glossary will serve as a valuable resource in navigating the world of pharmacology for everyday people.

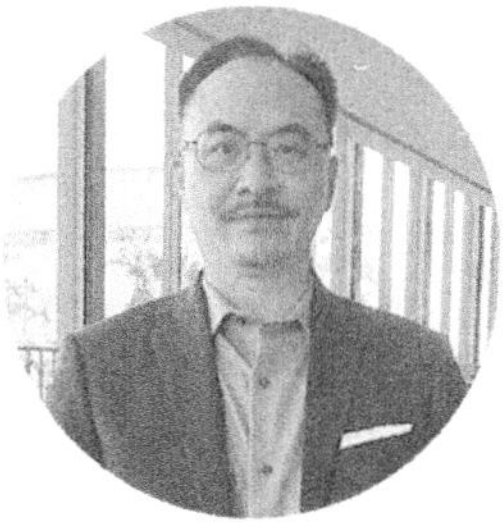

About the Author

Arthur Wang received a B.S. in Biochemistry from UCLA. He also had extensive studies in microbiology, immunology, western medicine, and traditional Chinese medicine. He is also an enthusiastic writer on various topics on the internet. Besides working, he has been actively involved in volunteer work for many years. Arthur Wang lives and works in Los Angeles, California.

Made in the USA
Monee, IL
04 November 2026

67378955R00079